"Throughout the U.S., there are significant disparities in Alzheimer's and dementia diagnosis rates, access to treatment, and quality care. But there don't have to be. In fact, we can begin to level the playing field right at home. Patricia Boswell's *Caregiving with Love and Joy* provides critical lessons and pertinent information that every family can utilize to better understand Alzheimer's disease and related dementias, and then create better, more meaningful daily interactions with those who are suffering."

—Goldie Byrd, PhD, executive director, Center for Outreach in Alzheimer's, Aging, and Community Health

"Patricia Boswell writes as if she is your warm and wise close friend, one who is a remarkably experienced nurse and caregiver. The book is full of practical knowledge and solutions for the many challenges of caregiving. I especially admire that Boswell starts with and frequently returns to the theme of self-care for the caregiver—this is the key to sustainable and loving care. Bravo for a book that will improve the lives of many caregivers and their loved ones!"

—Tia Powell, MD, professor of epidemiology and psychiatry, Albert Einstein College of Medicine; author of *Dementia Reimagined: Building a Life of Joy and Dignity from Beginning to End*

"From a public health perspective, few diseases are as devastating as dementia and Alzheimer's. Yet I have seen firsthand that having the right daily care can make all the difference in the long-term success of each patient. This book provides the simple and professional steps any family can implement to make the life of their loved one more comfortable, more enjoyable, and less stressful, which is the key to better outcomes."

—Takeisha C. Davis, MD, MPH, CEO, New Orleans East Hospital

Caregiving
with Love *and* Joy

AN EXPERT'S GUIDE TO PROVIDING THE BEST
ALZHEIMER'S DISEASE AND DEMENTIA HOME CARE

Patricia A. Boswell, LPN, MBA

AVERY
an imprint of Penguin Random House
New York

AVERY

An imprint of Penguin Random House LLC
penguinrandomhouse.com

Copyright © 2022 by Patricia Boswell and Pamela Liflander
Images © Gregory Jones, Jr.

ISBN (trade paperback) 9780593330692
ISBN (ebook) 9780593330708

Book design by Laura K. Corless

144555897

To my parents, James and Helen Boswell

Caring is daring.

Caring is understanding while sometimes being misunderstood.

For those who have taken on the rainbow of this task,
denial sits by us from time to time.

Yet the heart always attaches to the heart who needs us most.

While I may not always feel appreciated,
I will be present for you with love and joy.

CONTENTS

Contents

The Right Caregiver
Makes All the Difference

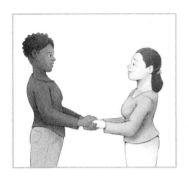

've always known that the right caregiver could make a difference, but I never thought it was a life-or-death decision until I had to force my way into my 82-year-old aunt's life to take care of her, almost five years after her diagnosis of Alzheimer's disease (AD). Even though my family knew full well that I was a home healthcare and hospice nurse, I wasn't asked to get involved until my aunt seemed to be on a total and complete downward spiral. The truth was, one of her sons, who lived close by, was in a deep state of denial and couldn't see how much help his mother really needed. The other son, who lived far away in Atlanta, finally intervened and contacted me out of desperation.

By the time my Atlanta cousin called me to intervene, my aunt was severely depressed, hallucinating, and unable to respond or engage in conversation. She had been in and out of the hospital six times over the previous year with urinary tract infections. Her new condominium wasn't fit for her to live in because her local son had never helped her unpack: she didn't have a proper couch or chair in the living room, or a decent table to take her meals. She was left to spend her days in a power bed watching television.

I started by straightening out her home and brought in the right furniture so that she would be safe and comfortable. This fix alone enabled her to get out of her bed and back to walking, which improved her mood. Then I had the kitchen and living room walls painted a cheerful yellow because it was her favorite color. In the bedroom I used a pale blue, which is thought to be calming for people with dementia. I decorated her bathroom in a darker blue so she would know that she was in a different room, and it would still have a soothing influence.

I asked to see her medical records, and found out that my local cousin wasn't keeping any, so I took out my LPN Daily Observation list and gave her a thorough exam. The first thing I noticed was her overgrown toenails. Toenails may not seem like a big issue, but I realized that if no one was monitoring her feet, it was quite likely that I would uncover other, more dangerous health issues brought on by a lack of care.

It took me five months to get my aunt back to real health and on a regular schedule of doctor appointments. I took her to see a podiatrist and found a primary care doctor who specialized in geriatric dementia care. She hadn't had a mammogram, chest X-ray, or MRI in years; her previous doctor hadn't recommended these tests because of her advanced age. Yet a mammogram showed that she had potentially cancerous nodules in her lymph nodes and needed to see an oncologist. If she hadn't had that mammogram, we would never have learned this information, and quite frankly, she might have died long ago.

It wasn't until my aunt was showing significant signs of improvement that I felt comfortable relinquishing my role and made her children, my cousins, the primary caregivers. By that point, I had cared for my aunt for three and a half years. I taught them the same instructions that are in this book. She was able to spend her last years looking and acting like a totally different person from the day I had appointed myself her guardian. Once she had access to the right foods, exercise, and activities, her mind was stronger. She was more resilient because her health and mood were under control.

I am a licensed practical nurse (LPN) who is on the front lines of caregiving every day. This story is just one of the hundreds I have lived through over the years working as a professional caregiver, a job that became even more complicated with COVID-19, and what the disease taught all of us about nursing home care. Since then, many families no longer want to put their loved ones in a facility or are afraid to have healthcare workers come into their homes. I don't blame them. But what that means is that we are all in the same boat. Whether you expected to be the primary caregiver or not, you are now. If you were able to hire help in the past, that luxury may be gone. If you were considering putting your mother, father, or grandparent in a nursing home, now rebranded as a skilled nursing inpatient facility (SNIF), you may want to think again. All across the country, most nursing homes are privately owned, and their owners have been getting away with understaffing for far too long. The employees are overworked and underpaid and are not always able to provide the very best care.

You may find yourself in this position for other reasons. No one wants, or expects, their loved ones to have AD or another form of dementia. These are devastating illnesses, to be sure. I'm here to tell you that caregiving will not be the end of your life as you know it. In fact, I truly believe that taking complete responsibility for someone you love, who has loved you all their life, can be one of the most rewarding parts of your life's journey. There will be days that are hard. And there will be many others that are so filled with joy that it cracks your heart open. My goal is to help you have as many of these wonderful, memorable days as possible.

MY STORY

The most rewarding part of my job has always been advocating for my clients. I love providing them with more opportunities than they or their families thought were possible, which leads to a better quality of life even as they decline. Yet the part of my job that has kept me most engaged over the years is listening to and learning from older people's stories.

I first recognized this passion when I was just about six years old. I lived across the street from a huge nursing home. Today, many nursing homes are more like detention facilities. But in those days, the seniors who lived there were encouraged to go outside by themselves and walk around the block. That was why I saw these elders all the time, and I liked being around them. I'm pretty outgoing, so I would make conversation. I would visit them, and sit down, and talk, and listen to their stories.

I also come from a family of nurses. In fact, I'm a third-generation nurse. My great-aunt was a nurse, and her niece (my aunt with dementia) was as well. Now we have doctors in the family, too, but when I was growing up, African American women were nurses. I passed the licensing exam to become an LPN when I was still in my nursing program, and then I transferred to business school. I was just one class short of getting my associate degree in nursing, but I wanted to try something new, so I applied and was offered a scholarship to Marymount Manhattan College to get my degree in business management.

When I graduated, I became a production supervisor for Avon

and stayed for almost nine years. I like to say that I use nursing in business and business in nursing, and it's true. Nursing taught me how to assess people. Nursing also teaches you how to be a good listener, because you have to be able to pick up cues from the patient in order to deliver the best care. Meanwhile, I quickly figured out that there aren't a lot of good listeners in the business world.

When my husband, Ronald, took a job as a college basketball coach at West Virginia University, I made the switch back to nursing and stayed in New York City. I had just had my first child, and nursing gave me the flexibility to raise a family and take time off in large chunks and travel from New York to West Virginia. The best nurses were the ones who could think like a businessperson: a problem solver. You need to be able to strategize, be results-oriented, and manage people. These three skills come together to alleviate stress for yourself, your patients, and their families, which leads to better health outcomes.

While I was working in nursing, providing end-of-life care for patients at home who were dying from the AIDS epidemic, I started my first company on the side. I wanted an all-natural laundry detergent that my whole family could use, including my baby, and I was surprised that there was nothing on the market that was exactly right. I knew from my time at Avon that the chemicals in adult detergents aren't really healthy for kids, and that I could do it better. My product, Safonique, was so successful that eventually Walmart picked it up, and running the brand became a full-time job for more than twenty years. I've always lived by the adage that when you want to get something done you find a busy woman, so I also received my MBA.

It wasn't until the 2008 recession that I went back to nursing again, and I've been working in this capacity ever since while continuing to run my business. By this time the medical industry had changed completely, and I had to pick a specialty. Remembering my comfort with older people, I chose geriatric and end-of-life care, and I never looked back. I love taking care of my patients and being their voice with doctors, healthcare providers, and sometimes their own families. The fact is, when people's minds are declining, they need someone not only to take care of them but to advocate for them.

Over the past twelve years, I've realized that I could help more people if I put my best practices down on paper. I know that I have real insight into how to get the best outcomes for my clients by providing the right care at the right time. Because I am both a businesswoman and a nurse, I do things a little differently. My techniques are efficient, empathetic, and results-oriented. My patients thrive because I care for them without creating additional stress or drama. While doctors provide excellent medical advice, they have no formal training in caregiving or how to address the often surprising behaviors that accompany dementia. Most cannot teach new caregivers how to best manage their days, make their home safe and comfortable, or deal with the physical and mental changes that come with this devastating diagnosis. And unless they have personal experience as a caregiver themselves, most doctors don't really know what it's like to live with someone with dementia. The truth is, individuals with dementia can live as long as twenty years after being diagnosed, and without the proper guidance, caregiving will lead to frustration, boredom, and worse, depression, for both you and your loved one.

I'm also in a unique position because I'm African American, and as far as I can tell, there are no dementia resources that directly address treating and caring for people of color. That's not to say that this book, and the lessons inside, are specific to a particular demographic. Taking care of my own is exactly the same as taking care of anyone else. However, I'm particularly interested in helping people of color because my people have been historically underserved by the medical community. I've watched too many people of color succumb to this disease in ways that they didn't have to.

For instance, I am certified as a clinical trial associate, which means that I am qualified to manage a clinical trial. If people of color understood the benefits of participating in clinical trials and tapping into other local, state, and federal resources that are available early on, their outcomes could be significantly better. The problem is that so many people don't think they're entitled to social services, or they think they're supposed to do everything on their own. They also are prone to wait to ask for help outside their immediate circle, by which time it's often too late to take advantage of what these clinical trials and social services can offer.

HOW THE BOOK WORKS

My goal is for you to have a positive caregiving experience. The key is to know how to provide exactly the right type of support so that your Loved One can stay in a private home: either yours or theirs. My aim is to take the fear out of caregiving and provide real-world advice from deep in the trenches. This book is also meant to answer the questions you may have that you have been afraid to ask, or that you don't know who to turn to or where to go for the right information. Read it straight through now, especially if your loved one is able to communicate. This way you can use the advice throughout to start the difficult conversations, especially about end-of-life decisions, so that you will be able to plan for the future. Then use the book as a reference, turning to the advice as you need it.

Part I is written just for you, the caregiver. You may have already read other books that are focused on the disease and the patient and address self-care as an afterthought. Yet I know that every caregiver is only at their best when they are tending to their needs as well. I always place self-care up front, so that you can adopt these crucial lessons before you develop habits that may negatively affect your own health and well-being.

First, you'll learn how to recognize typical dementia behaviors and why they often appear much earlier than you would think. The greatest obstacle that I see families face is denial, and I will help you push through and see your new reality and make the important decisions early. While no two cases of AD or dementia are the same, approaching the disease with eyes wide open is the one factor that may lead to a reversal of some health conditions that are associated with it, or, at the very least, a slowdown of progression. It also gives you the critical time you need to get everything you need in place.

The single most life-changing lesson is that the best caregivers are never in this battle alone. It is simply not possible to act like a superhero and save the day on your own. I show you how to form the optimal team that will help you take care of your loved one. Just like the Nigerian Igbo saying "It takes a village to raise a child," when it comes to AD and dementia, you will need to put together your own village of doctors, paraprofessionals, and others who will make your life easier and help you provide the best care.

Then I review self-care strategies so that you are taking care of yourself mentally, physically, and spiritually every day. My suggestions aren't rocket science, but just the knowledge that you have permission to spend some time every day on you is a lot more than most caregivers have. The worst thing that can happen to a caregiver is that they get sick and there is no one else available to take on their role. The second worst thing is burnout, which leads to anger, resentment, and frustration. Neither of those problems will happen if you take my advice.

The last chapter of Part I shows you exactly how to organize the home where you will be doing the caregiving. In the beginning of the disease, you may be living separately from your loved one and taking care of them for just a few hours a day. I have found that making small adjustments to their home as early as possible will make life for everyone infinitely easier. Many of these suggestions are safety tips, and I believe that you can never be too safe if you want your loved one to stay in their own home for as long as possible. I promise, the home we create together will not look or feel antiseptic, nor will it cost lots of money to fix up.

In Part II you will learn exactly what you need to know in order to provide optimal caregiving with love. Our loved ones with dementia need to participate in activities that will keep them engaged and active. They deserve to be treated with respect and compassion and feel that they are in control of their lives with the ability to make choices. In short, they need to feel as if they are succeeding, and to focus on what they can do rather than on what they can't. The reason is simple: when they experience success, they will stay calm, which makes your job 100 percent easier.

The next chapter is filled with tips and tricks that only the best-trained caregivers know so that you are no longer in a response mode and are operating more proactively. By using them every day, I experience less burnout in my own job and enjoy my time with my clients rather than becoming physically and emotionally drained.

Chapter 6 outlines what I do best: the day-to-day business of caregiving. I share basic nursing skills that are easy to master and over time will become second nature. Next, you'll learn how to deal with difficult behaviors, which is where people with dementia/AD get the worst rap. In reality, the way you communicate with your Loved One will make all the difference in their behavior. In order to communicate more effectively, you'll learn how to hold on to a positive mindset through the hard days. This is something that cannot be faked.

You will become an expert in identifying and treating common medical problems, and I share how they manifest in people with dementia. The best way to do this is to address symptoms on a daily basis. One of my tricks is to always work from a checklist, what I call the Daily Observation. This is a simple tool that enables you to notice and then track even the subtlest changes in health.

Chapter 9 covers the relationship between nutrition and health. For people with dementia/AD, this begins with making simple foods your loved one will enjoy eating and then ensuring that they actually eat. I also address issues surrounding food insecurity and food availability and teach you how to make the most nutritious food choices given limited options.

Lastly, we can face end-of-life decision-making with clarity and perspective. You will learn how to separate the denial and emotional response in order to make the most informed medical and financial plan. Hopefully you will not need to read this chapter for a long time. Yet if you are caring for someone at the end of their life, having a plan ensures that everyone has enough time to create positive lasting memories that are not tied to financial trauma or stress.

Caregiving for someone with dementia/AD can be a long haul. So that's why I'm here, helping you navigate. And I'm glad you're here. We're in this together.

PART I

Get Ready to Be the Best Caregiver

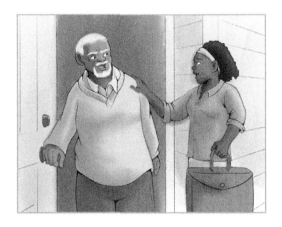

CHAPTER 1

Is This Behavior Normal?
Accepting the New Reality

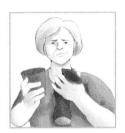

About twenty years ago I noticed that one of my neighbors, Kendra, was writing names and phone numbers on pieces of paper and taping them to the back of her bedroom door. I remember thinking at the time that it was odd, but it wasn't odd enough to bring it to the attention of her daughter and my friend, Alicia. Even though I am a nurse, I figured that those Post-it notes were her business, and I shouldn't get involved.

Two to three months later, though, it became clear that Kendra was changing. She was forgetful, repeating conversations, and making critical mistakes in the kitchen where she used to have total domination. Once, when we had stopped by for a visit, I noticed that she had left the water running in the sink. Another time I found a burnt and ruined teapot in the garbage can. She would shrug off these behaviors when I pointed them out, and frankly, I didn't want to get into a fight. The last straw was when she put a rug in the oven and almost set fire to the house. At that point it didn't take a nursing degree to see that this woman had dementia.

After what we have come to call "the rug incident," I told Alicia that it would be in her best interest to hold a family meeting with her relatives to figure out a plan. Yet they never did it. Why? Alicia and her siblings were in denial. They couldn't come to terms with the idea that their mother was less than perfectly healthy. They couldn't separate the reality of what was happening right in front of their eyes with their own life and their old familial roles. So even though my neighbor was clearly exhibiting the signs and symptoms of dementia, her children couldn't or didn't want to accept what they were seeing. Their reasoning was that "Mom's just getting old."

Luckily, I knew better, and within a week I was able to put in place a strategy for getting Kendra the coverage she needed and keeping her in her home. I made sure she knew that *we knew* her mental health was failing, and that we would work together to go forward successfully. Once we implemented a plan, she was able to relax knowing that her family supported her.

Kendra lived for another twenty years, in her own home, before she passed away. Those years were challenging and beautiful. Her family learned to work like a team, for her sake as well as theirs, since they shared the responsibility of being her caregiver. Today they would tell anyone who asked that the hardest work involved moving out of denial.

DENIAL IS SAFE

Maybe you bought this book because you have a concern, a gut feeling that something is going on with someone you love. It could be your parent, spouse, close friend, or relative. It may even be your adult child. Just taking this one step and buying this book means that you are already coming out of denial. Denial is when a person is faced with a fact that is too uncomfortable to accept, and so they reject the fact, even in the face of overwhelming evidence. When it comes to dementia, your Loved One (let's refer to this person as LO for short) may be in denial, because they are ashamed of how they are changing. The family may be in denial because they are afraid of the vulnerability this disease brings up. Denial is also influenced by what the diagnosis would mean to the whole family: an upheaval in everyone's life. You may be heartbroken when you see your LO struggling, which causes denial to look a lot like grief.

There are lots of reasons why denial and dementia are so closely tied together. Dementia is a sneaky, insidious disease. The symptoms come along so slowly that you may not notice them in real time, even if you're living with the person. And if you live far away from your LO and only see them from time to time, they may be hiding their symptoms or may have developed compensating behaviors. That's why my neighbor had all those Post-it notes: she knew that she was having a hard time remembering phone numbers, but she didn't want anyone else to know.

It's only when the compensation strategies no longer work that you may notice odd behaviors, and at this point another type of denial sets in. By this time, the excuses come fast. Some people don't want to see their LO not feeling well. I've heard too many times, "Mom's just getting old." I also know that lots of people get old and don't get dementia.

Denial is also influenced by the relationship someone has with the person they will have to care for. For instance, if you are harboring anger toward your parent, your denial may feel different than that of someone who has a strong attachment or closeness. Denial with anger may cause you to act out, or yell when they do something out of the ordinary (like deciding to dry a rug in the oven). If you find that you're getting agitated because your LO just asked the same question three times in a row, ask yourself why are *you* so angry.

Seeing your LO acting out of character may also bring up feelings of guilt, especially if you are in denial. Or you may have guilt that your relationship isn't as strong or as healthy as you want it to be. It's okay to feel guilty; we all do from time to time. It's not okay to let your guilt keep you from taking the next step. When you flip feelings of guilt into real concern, you move out of stagnancy and into a more proactive mindset. And proactive is the place you need to be.

Denial also comes from confusion when you are feeling overwhelmed or lost. This is not surprising for a first-time caregiver; you can't imagine the changes that are to come or what exactly you will need to do. You may feel like you are in shock now, yet when you look back, the dementia signs were there all along. Luckily, I'm here to help ease this confusion. You will be able to count on the knowledge I've gained from experience as you move forward in your new role.

No matter how you feel about your LO, the sooner you get past denial, the better. It not only alleviates wasted time in terms of providing better care, it gives you more time to come up with strategies that work for you. The time you are going to spend caregiving is time you cannot ever get back. The good news is that once everyone is out of denial, a family can move toward acceptance, and with that comes relief. Best of all, that mindset comes with better health outcomes for your LO, and a better caregiving experience for you.

THE SIGNS AND SYMPTOMS OF DEMENTIA: EXACTLY WHAT AM I LOOKING FOR?

The single thing that's going to get you and your family out of denial is understanding the behaviors that you're seeing. We all experience memory lapses: forgetting a friend's name during a conversation, or walking into a room and wondering why you are there. These blips may be caused by anxiety, a bad night's sleep (or a few in a row), illness, a new medication, poor diet, or dealing with physical pain. When you notice that someone's memory lapses interfere with their ability to get through the day, or continue for days at a time, it's possibly a greater problem. I tell the families of my patients that dementia isn't when you can't find your keys. It's forgetting what keys are for. Before we get into the signs of dementia, here's a list of what it is, and what it is not:

Dementia is . . .	Dementia is not . . .
Consistently poor judgment and decision-making	Making a bad decision once in a while
Inability to manage a budget, overspending, or consistent financial errors	Missing a single monthly payment
Losing track of the date or the season	Forgetting which day it is, but remembering it later
Difficulty participating in a conversation	Difficulty remembering the right word or name in the moment, but remembering it later
Finding objects in inappropriate places, like finding knives in the freezer	Difficulty remembering where you put something down
Getting lost in a familiar place	Using GPS or Google Maps to get home from a place you've been to once or twice before
Wearing two different shoes, or wearing shoes on the wrong foot	Misplacing shoes

Dementia and AD have early warning signs and symptoms, but because they are so subtle, family members often miss them, refuse to accept them, or hide the fact that they've noticed something strange because they don't want to intrude or say something that would be upsetting. Any one of these signs should be cause for immediate concern, and is enough to warrant taking your LO to a doctor for a diagnosis.

1. Adopting inappropriate behaviors: talking loudly, throwing tantrums, cursing
2. Changes in diet/eating habits
3. Difficulty completing sequential tasks: inability to drive a car after years of driving
4. Difficulty with *executive function*, including reasoning, problem solving, planning: this can show up during activities like grocery shopping, making doctor appointments, paying bills or cashing checks, or impulsive online shopping
5. Difficulty with visual and spatial awareness: a loss of depth perception may lead to falls and car accidents because of an increase in making abrupt moves while driving
6. Failure to recognize common objects: this decline can affect the cleanliness of the home
7. Visual hallucinations: reporting seeing people, animals, or even shapes or colors that do not exist
8. Lack of motivation and initiation: changes in mood, personality, or hygiene
9. Loss of focus and perceptual ability: losing the skills to finish a favorite activity
10. Loss of risk awareness, poor judgment: leaving credit cards at restaurants or stores
11. Personality and mood changes, including depression, increased anxiety, paranoia
12. Problems with orientation: getting lost while walking/driving to a familiar location
13. Repetitive questioning and storytelling
14. Withdrawal from work, family, or social activities
15. Obsessive-compulsive behaviors: detrimentally focusing intently on one activity

The importance of knowing these signs goes beyond identifying dementia. Let's take a lack of hygiene as an example. You may have noticed that your LO has a strong smell, their clothing is in poor shape when they used to be dressed to the nines, or they're wearing the same thing day after day. These signs may seem innocuous, but they can quickly lead to a decline in health with real ramifications. When women stop showering, for example, they are more likely to develop dangerous urinary tract infections. What's more, one small symptom may be a signal of more than one of the "official" warning signs. If your LO isn't changing their clothing daily, they may have also stopped seeing their friends. Or they may be having trouble with buttons or zippers, signs of incoordination.

It's also possible that your LO doesn't know that they are struggling. In fact, this is another form of denial. I've met lots of dementia patients who will tell me that their memory is just fine. I've learned over the years that it's the exception for someone with dementia to complain about their memory. (Doctors often say that if someone complains about their memory, they are more likely to be stressed, anxious, or depressed.) So, when you see these signs and symptoms for your LO, you are experiencing their life entirely differently than they are.

HOW TO START DIFFICULT CONVERSATIONS

All of these should be a face-to-face conversation, even if it has to be over something like Zoom or FaceTime. The best case would be a neutral environment, not your home or theirs, and try to keep the conversation as casual as possible. Be kind and not confrontational.

> ## When Your LO Won't Go to the Doctor
>
> It's quite possible that your LO believes they are perfectly fine, even when you and the rest of your family see otherwise. One way to snap them out of denial is to get a formal evaluation from their doctor. But what happens if your LO refuses to go for the checkup? Luckily, there is a fix: telehealth. Your doctor can come to you via video calls or telehealth. What's more, the doctors you need your LO to see have dealt with this issue before, and their office is likely to have other solutions to suggest. Don't let stubbornness stand in the way of getting the medical care your LO deserves.

If this is your close friend, sibling, or parent in whom you've noticed changes even if you don't see them every day, you can say,

"I noticed last time I was in your home that you had a bunch of Post-it notes with phone numbers and names by the kitchen table. Did you forget how to find them in your contacts in your cell phone?" or *"I've noticed over the last couple of months that you are repeating stories to me about things we've already talked about. Have you picked up on that, too?"* or *"I noticed when we went out for dinner last night that you were staring at the menu for a long time and had difficulty understanding the headings, even though you've been to that restaurant a million times. Is everything okay?"*

If this is your spouse, whom you see every day, say,

"I think it's time to see a doctor to check out your memory." Or "Yesterday you didn't put the milk back in the refrigerator and I found it in the

pantry this morning. The same thing happened last week. Let's get to the bottom of this because I'm concerned about you."

If you are concerned about a casual friend or a distant family member, approach someone else in their family and say,

"You know, I'm concerned about your sister. Last time we had lunch she couldn't remember how she got to the restaurant and seemed confused. I think you should take her to be evaluated by a doctor. This isn't normal behavior."

If this is a colleague at work, talk to their manager and say,

"Tom seems to be struggling with his assignment and it's holding back my work. I've noticed several signs that may be pointing to memory loss. He's confused about deadlines and the projects he's working on. Can you have a conversation with him?"

Don't be surprised if you get pushback and denial. Most people with dementia think they're fine. Respond by saying,

"I know you think you're fine, but I'm worried about you. We need to see the doctor to make me feel better. It may be nothing, or it may be something. I'm going to make the appointment."

WHAT'S HAPPENING INSIDE THE DEMENTIA/AD BRAIN

Dementia is a progressive brain disease, which means that it will get worse over time. It slowly destroys a person's memory and, along with that, it inhibits learning new skills or maintaining ones they already have. It affects one's ability to understand, reason, and make good decisions. These are often referred to as *cognitive symptoms*. Often, these cognitive symptoms occur when the person is in otherwise excellent health, and they can even happen before midlife.

How dementia begins is not entirely understood. The latest research points to a few distinct mechanisms that occur in the brain and cause memory loss. For some people, the brain stops receiving enough fuel from the foods we eat to make it run quickly and efficiently. That fuel comes in the form of glucose, which the body converts from carbohydrate-rich foods. This disconnection between the brain and diet is one reason why some doctors refer to AD as type 3 diabetes.

We also know that some dementias affect the brain from the outside in: from the outer brain lobes to the core. And depending on the area of the brain that's affected, dementia can present in a different way from one person to the next. The frontal lobes control behaviors, planning, and decision-making. As you move closer to the midbrain, the parietal lobes control body functions and movement. The last part of the brain to be affected is the temporal lobes, which hold memory and language.

IS IT ALZHEIMER'S DISEASE
OR ANOTHER TYPE OF DEMENTIA?

Dementia is the broad category that covers the loss of memory and other cognitive abilities to the extent that they interfere with everyday life. There are many types of dementia, and they are grouped by what they have in common, such as the part of the brain that's affected. See your LO's primary care physician first: they will provide the initial diagnosis. Then they should recommend that your LO see a neurologist, who will identify which type of dementia your LO has, or if their memory problems are related to something else, like depression, medication side effects, or addiction to drugs or alcohol. Regardless of what type of dementia your LO has, the way you will care for them will be the same. Right now, there is no cure for dementia of any kind. The best we can do is slow the progression through medications and the behavioral interventions that come from excellent care.

Alzheimer's disease is the most common form of dementia. It typically occurs with plaques and tangles developing in the brain that block the brain's ability to access memories, including the memory of physical processes. This process of brain and bodily forgetting is referred to as *retrogenesis*, a return to childhood. Unfortunately, these tangles and plaques are only identified on autopsy: there is no test for Alzheimer's disease, which is why most people who have dementia are put in this category.

Vascular dementia is the second most common type of dementia, caused by damage to the blood vessels in the brain. This damage blocks brain cells from receiving oxygen and other nutrients. Vascular dementia often occurs after a stroke. Symptoms include difficulty with problem solving, slower thinking, and loss of focus and organization.

Lewy body dementia presents with distinct symptoms. People with Lewy body dementia are known to act out their dreams during sleep, have visual hallucinations, have difficulty with focus and attention, and have tremors and rigidity similar to Parkinson's disease.

Frontotemporal dementia is characterized by changes to one's personality, behavior, and language, which are all controlled in the frontal lobes of the brain.

Huntington's disease is a progressive brain disorder caused by a genetic mutation. This disease has a very early onset—between ages 30 and 40—and results in limited movement, mood destabilization, and diminished thinking skills.

Creutzfeldt-Jakob disease is an extremely rare genetic disease that may also be caused by exposure to diseased nervous system tissue, such as from an organ transplant. As brain cells are destroyed, the damage that results leads to a rapid decline in thinking, muscle movements, difficulty walking, and mood changes.

The Activities of Daily Living (ADLs)

Your LO will need some form of caregiving when they are no longer able to complete each of these tasks on their own. They are also a measure of when someone qualifies for government assistance through Medicare and Medicaid:

- Personal hygiene: bathing/showering, grooming, nail care, brushing teeth
- Toileting and continence: ability to control bladder and bowel functions, get to and from the toilet, and clean oneself
- Dressing: the ability to put on and take off clothing as well as make appropriate decisions based on weather/occasion
- Eating: the ability to eat and to prepare simple meals
- Transferring: the ability to go from sitting to standing, as well as getting in and out of bed and walking from one location to another

A WINDOW OF HOPE:
SOME DEMENTIAS CAN BE REVERSED

Sometimes memory loss can result from other causes besides dementia. In fact, many people experiencing dementia-like symptoms may achieve a complete return to good health once an accurate diagnosis is made, followed by the right kinds of treatment. In my experience, roughly 10 percent of people with dementia-like symptoms do not in fact have dementia and have other conditions that are reversible.

These health issues include the following:

Depression/anxiety: A specific incident, a loss, or stress can make someone seem forgetful or like they are "losing their mind." These symptoms come on suddenly and can resolve once the person learns better coping strategies. In contrast, dementia and AD develop over time and do not resolve with behavioral therapeutic approaches.

Alcohol/substance abuse: Constant alcohol use prevents the body from properly processing vitamin B1, which is linked to dementia. This may be why alcoholics and drug users often have gaps in long-term memory, lie to fill in those gaps, and struggle to learn new information. These complaints may resolve once the person stops abusing these substances.

Infections and immune disorders: Something as ordinary as a high fever or urinary tract infection can cause dementia symptoms. What's more, the medications that treat infections can cause dementia-like symptoms, too.

Nutritional and/or hormone irregularities: Those with thyroid problems; low blood sugar; dehydration; or too little sodium, calcium, copper, or vitamins B and D often develop dementia symptoms or personality changes, which can be reversed by changing one's diet.

Subdural hematomas: Bleeding between the brain and the skull following a fall or a concussion can cause dementia symptoms, which will reverse after healing.

Let's Start Record Keeping

One of the cornerstones of professional nursing is learning how to assess any situation and to keep detailed notes. If you are worried that your LO is exhibiting signs of dementia, it's time to start record keeping. Find an empty journal or binder (which you will soon learn is invaluable) and write down your observations.

Start by answering these questions:

1. What's different about my LO's behavior? What are they doing or not doing that is a cause for concern? Has anyone else noticed odd behaviors? Who are the likely people I should follow up with?
2. What other health issues are they dealing with, and are those issues making the dementia symptoms worse?
3. What lifestyle issues are they dealing with, and are those issues making the dementia symptoms worse?
4. Who is the best person to approach my LO with my concerns, and where/when should the conversation take place?
5. Who is the best choice to accompany my LO to the doctor for the initial evaluation?

Toxins: Significant exposure to heavy metals like lead in drinking water, mercury in fish and dental fillings, and pesticides may cause dementia symptoms.

Brain tumors: Although rare, these tumors affect thinking and personality.

THE STAGES OF DEMENTIA/AD

Dementia and AD are typically described as having seven phases/stages, but I think it's easier to group them into three categories: mild, moderate, and severe. Most people follow their own slow, progressive trajectory: they move from one stage to the next, the speed of which can be influenced by the quality of care they receive. Some resources say that the average person with AD lives four to eight years past their diagnosis. However, if you catch the disease in the early, mild stages and begin to provide exceptional care, your LO can live with Alzheimer's for as long as twenty years. Either way, it's best to understand this trajectory as early as possible. The more you know, the better you can plan and prepare for the later, more challenging stages.

What's more, for many of those years they will not require significant caregiving. The earliest stages of dementia may simply involve supervision and encouragement as they continue to live their lives. The middle stages will require more hands-on participation by caregivers in order to preserve a safe and desirable quality of life. The final stages will require caregivers to provide the most active care and comfort.

EARLY OR MILD DEMENTIA/AD

Stage 1—No Cognitive Decline: A doctor may refer to this stage as "preclinical" because there are no symptoms. If your LO's family has a history of dementia/AD, their doctor may interview them about memory problems as part of their regular physical. This means that your LO may know that they are in this stage but isn't sharing that information. This stage may last for years or decades and is the most important period in which preventive measures like improving diet and increasing exercise can affect the progression of the disease.

Stage 2—Very Mild Cognitive Decline: At this point what may have seemed like normal forgetfulness is more concerning to the individual, because they have noticed a steeper decline in cognitive functioning. This is the stage where your LO may create compensating strategies like list making or relying on their calendar so that their decline is less noticeable and won't interfere with work or socializing. Some compensating strategies are so effective that you may not notice any difference at all, or simply think that "Mom is getting older." You may remember one time Dad did something strange, but the single incidents aren't adding up to be a big problem. Doctors often refer to this stage as mild cognitive impairment or MCI.

Stage 3—Mild Cognitive Decline: By this point a person's forgetfulness may become apparent to a keen observer. You may notice that your LO is having difficulty concentrating, takes longer to accomplish everyday tasks, or told you about getting lost going to a favorite location. They may have a harder time remembering the right words or names in a conversation, or become distraught when a valuable object, like a favorite piece of jewelry, has been misplaced. They may no longer be able to manage their personal finances—by forgetting to pay bills, getting sucked into a telephone scam, and so on—or go to the grocery store by themselves.

Stage 3 is often the time when individuals are first evaluated by a doctor, especially if there was no family history of dementia/AD. It is also the stage where denial becomes a flashpoint between family members. It is also the most reasonable time to form an action plan. A person can maintain Stage 3 for as long as seven years without requiring full-time caregiving. At this point meals should be provided, as your LO should no longer cook for themselves (for safety reasons). They will need frequent check-ins and daily visits if they are living alone. If you notice the physical signs mentioned earlier, they may require help with some but not all of the ADLs.

MIDDLE OR MODERATE DEMENTIA/AD

Stage 4—Moderate Cognitive Decline: The middle stages of dementia/ AD go quickly. Stage 4 lasts about two years and is the most likely point at which you'll receive a firm diagnosis. By now, your LO's compensation strategies are no longer effective, and their work life suffers. They may get into a car accident because they misjudged their speed or the speed of other cars, after which they should no longer be driving. Reading the newspaper may become frustrating because they can't hold on to whatever they just read. You may notice that your LO is withdrawing from family events or socializing with friends because engaging with others is becoming problematic, or they are ashamed of having inappropriate outbursts of anger or using vulgar language. They have trouble with the ADLs and require more than a daily check-in to help with meal preparation or to accompany them to a doctor appointment. By this point your LO can no longer be left alone.

Stage 5—Moderately Severe Cognitive Decline: This stage is also likely to last for two years, and by the end your LO will require significant support for many hours each day. Memory loss has begun to affect all facets of life, including most of the ADLs. Your LO may forget the names of distant family members or the details of major events. These inabilities cause frustration, anger, and suspiciousness. They may have hallucinations or delusions.

LATE OR SEVERE DEMENTIA/AD

Stage 6—Severe Cognitive Decline: The later stages of dementia/AD can last a long time if your LO is otherwise in good health. Typically, Stage 6 lasts for more than two years. People in this stage may recall long-term memories, such as childhood or the teenage years, while having little or no short-term memory, including the names of close family members. Caregiving support should include helping your LO with eating, dressing, hygiene, and toileting. They will no longer be able to count backward from the number ten, and some people begin to stutter. Dealing with these losses can cause deep states of depression. They may also start to sleep more during the day and become confused or wander in the late afternoon/early evening. This behavior is called *sundowning*.

Stage 7—Very Severe Cognitive Decline: The length of this stage depends on your LO's health outside of dementia/AD and the quality of care they are receiving. However, once it starts, it's a precipitous decline to end of life. By this point a person with dementia/AD often cannot speak or communicate their needs. They may be unable to sit up on their own or hold their head up, and they may be prone to having seizures. Their body becomes more rigid and they experience pain; they may even hold a grim expression rather than a smile. They will regress to more infantile behaviors like sucking, and sleep for long periods during the day. They are typically less agitated and, in many ways, easier to care for, although they require more "heavy lifting" as they become immobile. Difficulty eating typically leads to significant dehydration and weight loss. Limited mobility increases the risk of bedsores and skin infections. These physical conditions are the typical causes of death. As you'll learn, it is possible to keep your LO at home, under your care, through Stage 7, and we'll discuss how to tap into all kinds of services to make this situation more manageable.

ACCEPTING THE NEW NORMAL

Working in home healthcare, I've seen hundreds of sick, elderly, and frail individuals refuse to give up control because they haven't accepted that their mind and body are changing. More tragically, I continually find that my clients' LOs haven't thought through how a dementia/AD diagnosis will change everyone's life. The truth is, this diagnosis isn't just applicable to the person with the disease; everyone around them will be affected.

If you were able to identify the signs of the early stages, consider yourself lucky. You still have time on your side to work with your LO and come up with strategies and plans for the future that work for everyone involved. These will help prepare you for the later stages, and you can implement some right now. I guarantee your life will be easier in the long run.

However, if your LO is already in a middle or moderate stage, you may have more challenges to deal with. First, you have to come to terms with the fact that your LO is no longer the same person they used to be. Your family's job is to learn how to love and accept this person for who they are *now*. In order to do that, you need to accept the switch in roles that accompanies this diagnosis: You may be a child caring for your parents, or a spouse responsible for the care of a previously independent partner. You may have to put your career, retirement, or vacation plans on hold until you work out a way forward. However, this role reversal doesn't have to be for the worse. In fact, it may even deepen your relationship.

YOU ARE NOT ALONE

Forget what you have heard from friends or seen on television. Caregiving does not have to be lonely, frustrating, or depressing. As the number of people with dementia/AD grows, so does the community of caregivers. In fact, according to the National Alliance for Caregiving and AARP, there are more than 16 million dementia/AD caregivers in the United States right now.[1] That means that there is no better time to make new friends or find support through a group in your town or online. Both AARP (www.aarp.org) and the Alzheimer's Association (www.alz.org) offer opportunities for caregivers to get together, share triumphs, and learn strategies for making everyone's lives easier.

Remember, anyone can be a great caregiver. While most are women, people from all age, racial, and ethnic groups; income and educational levels; gender identities; and sexual orientations take on this responsibility. If you stay open to the idea that the new normal is just another challenge—one that you can conquer with the right tools and support—you will have a much easier time transitioning into the role.

This is particularly true for people of color. I have found that Black and Brown families are often reluctant to put their aging LOs in nursing homes and are left to provide caregiving themselves. Dealing with dementia/AD is no exception. In fact, statistically there are more Black and Brown folks dealing with dementia than any other racial demographic. According to a 2018 report from the Alzheimer's Association, African Americans are twice as likely to develop AD and other dementias, and Hispanics are 1.5 times as likely compared to White people in the United States.

Families of color often have a distrust of others outside the community, particularly in the medical profession, and often rely on generational living. This arrangement leaves the responsibility of care squarely on the shoulders of family members. According to a 2020 study from AARP, African American caregivers provide the most hours of care each week—31.2 hours on average—with Hispanic caregivers at 26.0 hours per week, significantly more than White caregivers.[2]

No matter what your family looks like, when your LO displays the symptoms of dementia, please quickly accept them as fact. Then use this book as a guide so that your LO receives the best possible care right in their own home.

Over the years, I've seen that caregivers seem to be getting younger. According to the same AARP report, 58 percent of caregivers are considered Gen X, Millennials, or Gen Z. This means that you may have responsibilities for your spouse and children as well as your parents. Take my friend Dominique, whose husband, Ernest, was the primary caregiver for his mother, who had dementia. About five years in, I noticed that whenever I saw Ernest around the neighborhood, something didn't seem quite right. Dominique would tell me that he was fine, just stressed out from taking care of his mother on his own. Ernest's brothers weren't helping out, and the sons refused to put her in a memory care center.

This conversation went on for about two years. Then, just a few months later, Dominique called to tell me that Ernest had been diagnosed with early-onset dementia. And at age 64, he was actually diagnosed in a later stage than his mother. Luckily, Dominique didn't fall into the trap of denial this time. She knew that she wasn't strong enough physically to take care of both Ernest and his mother by herself. So she asked their adult daughter, Kelsey, to come to the rescue. At 47, Kelsey has moved into the house to be the primary caregiver for both her father and her grandmother.

WHAT'S NEXT

Now that you have a better understanding of what your LO is experiencing and what the future may hold, it's time to start mastering the art of caregiving. The rest of the book contains everything you will need to know to get through each day with grace and dignity, no matter what stage of dementia your LO is in.

The secret to a thriving caregiving experience is accepting that you have specific needs, wants, and desires that can and should be met. While other "experts" may say that you should take your LO into account first, I believe that you should operate from a mindset that takes you, your life, and the rest of your family into consideration with every decision. The best way to do that is to recognize that you are not on this journey alone. In the next chapter, we will brainstorm an ideal team of supporters and real experts who will be integral in helping you provide exceptional care every day.

CHAPTER 2

Becoming the Best Caregiver

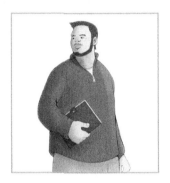

The first big decision any family with a dementia/AD diagnosis faces is *"Who will be the primary caregiver?"* Even if your LO is in the earliest stages of the disease, it's important to start these discussions as a family in preparation for what is to come.

The primary caregiver has many roles, including coordinating the LO's mental and physical care. The primary caregiver is also the team's leader, the medical record keeper, and the LO's most frequent companion.

Considering the very idea of being a caregiver can seem daunting. Many people don't feel that they have the necessary skills and knowledge to be prepared. However, what makes for an exceptional caregiver is not scientific knowledge or superhuman strength. The best caregivers I've met are patient, organized, and flexible. They are also good communicators and managers and maintain a positive attitude even when things don't go as planned. If you have any of these traits and the time and the financial ability to be a caregiver, it can be a very rewarding experience. What's more, you'll be able to carry over the lessons you'll learn into other parts of your life.

The specific day-to-day caregiving skills can be acquired and developed "on the job." First, you need to learn about the many facets of this disease. This book will help; I also recommend spending time on the Alzheimer's Association website, as it offers an excellent primer. Having a full understanding of what to look for and expect will help you talk to your LO's doctor intelligently and understand what they are saying. It will also help you explain what your LO is experiencing on the day-to-day level.

Excellent caregivers know how to:

- Access resources
- Administer medications
- Arrange transportation
- Interpret what your LO is trying to communicate
- Make decisions and take action
- Manage the household: paying bills, cleaning the home, and creating a safe and sustainable environment
- Monitor your LO's daily health
- Negotiate the healthcare system
- Offer companionship
- Plan and provide meals
- Provide emotional support
- Provide hands-on care

Does My Loved One Want Me?

Sometimes the LO self-selects a caregiver within the family and develops a close relationship with that person in an effort to groom them. However, they may not be the best choice—perhaps they're not a good personality match for caregiving, or they don't live close enough and aren't willing to move. Even in the earliest stages, the primary caregiver should live no more than 20 to 30 minutes away, because they will have to make regular accommodations to the LO's home, or their own.

I always say *If you see something, say something.* When a family I know had to choose a caregiver and health proxy, the father chose his oldest son, even though one of his daughters was a nurse: they had a perfect choice with a capable healthcare professional, but he chose the son simply because he was oldest. This decision created problems every time the father needed medical care, because the daughter, who could make insightful recommendations, was constantly left out of the conversation. I suggested to the daughter that she hold a family meeting to discuss a better way forward, and the son agreed that his sister was a better choice. Their father was able to change his mind when he realized that his son was comfortable giving up this role—and even relieved. Then, as a family, they decided to make the daughter the primary caregiver.

THE INITIAL ASSESSMENT: KNOW YOUR LO

I was trained as a nurse to start every patient relationship with an assessment so that I fully understood the situation and could make the necessary plans for exceptional care. This includes evaluating both mental and physical health. As a family member, start the assessment process as soon as you spot behavioral changes. Assessment is the flip side of denial: you can't "unsee" what you have assessed.

Your initial assessment will be confirmed by your LO's doctor. Then you will assess your LO frequently, depending on the stage of dementia/AD they are in. In the early stages, caregiving may only mean a daily check-in. In the moderate stages, you will need to be present and available daily. This still may not mean that you are living together. Depending on their needs, you may have to stop in on your way to or from work. You may hire nighttime coverage or find someone to keep your LO company during the day if they are lonely. Making decisions on how much caregiving you need to provide will depend on your most recent assessment. Stay on the lookout for new signs and symptoms, adverse events, and positive responses to treatment.

In order to do a proper assessment, you also have to know who your LO is on an entirely new level than how you know them right now. You will have to learn their likes, dislikes, and past experiences. They may have experienced traumatic events that are reflected in present behaviors. For instance, someone who experienced suffering as a child may be angrier and unable to control their moods when they have dementia. Or they may have hallucinations that refer back to terrible memories.

The best way to gather this information is to spend time together outside the caregiving relationship, meaning not while you are tending to their needs. Going through photo albums, listening to music together, and reminiscing about other family members are good ways to get information. You can also assign another family member to be the "historian" and uncover this information for you.

I've also found that when you deliver culturally appropriate care, everyone benefits, whether that's through the meals you cook or the way you talk to their friends. Understanding where they come from will also give you a better idea about who you're taking care of and what really matters to them in terms of their traditions, history, values, and family systems. You may not embrace church services or be particularly religiously observant, but if your LO is, you need to include church and church activities as part of your caregiving.

Culture may even express itself in more nuanced ways among family members. My friend Paula has a son, Clarence, who is dating Jun, who is from China. If Jun had to be a caregiver for Paula, the caregiving decisions she would make would be influenced by her own Chinese culture, even though Paula isn't Chinese. Jun and Clarence would have to come to an agreement on which of Jun's and Clarence's own cultural practices best serve Paula.

And when it comes to food, regional influences can be just as important as ethnic ones. My family comes from New Orleans, and we were brought up to eat red beans and rice every Monday for dinner, no matter who you are. That's culture within a culture. My husband's family comes from another part of the South, and that wasn't part of his upbringing. So if I ever need caregiving, I would want him (or another caregiver) to remember that's what I expect for dinner on Monday nights.

Factors That May Affect Dementia/AD

- Age
- Culture
- Current general health
- Education
- Family health history
- Geographic location
- Lifestyle
- Previous abilities and skills
- Previous health conditions
- Previous history with trauma or abuse
- Previous occupation
- Resiliency
- Standard of living

THE SIGNS OF ELDER ABUSE

You may have become a caregiver because you noticed that your LO was no longer able to care for themselves. Or you may be taking over for someone else who was not doing a great job. This often happens when a relative can't get past their familial role of deferring to their elders, no matter how much their behaviors are poorly influencing their well-being. While it may be upsetting to see that your LO isn't eating or bathing or changing their clothes, not addressing these issues is actually a lack of care, which is a form of elder abuse.

For instance, I once went to work for a family where the niece was the primary caregiver. When I walked into the house I was appalled: it was a pigsty. It turned out that the niece, who had been caring for her mother for ten years, had become a hoarder, packing the house with her own stuff. In this instance, the niece was making it more challenging for her aunt to live safely in her home by neglecting the house itself.

These signs may point to neglect or abuse by another caregiver. If you notice any of them, you're already on your way to being an exceptional caregiver:

- Dehydration
- Fear of previous caretaker
- Inadequate heating or cooling in the home
- Injuries, burns, bruises, or open sores
- Malnutrition
- Poor personal hygiene
- Prescription medications unfilled or expired, or signs of over-medication
- Unclean clothes or bedding

THE CAREGIVER'S BEST FRIEND: THE BINDER

The binder or journal you started in Chapter 1 will be your best friend and the key to your success. You are officially the librarian for your LO's medical records, and you need to understand every aspect of their mental and physical health so that you can communicate with their doctors and specialists. By keeping these notes in a physical binder or on your computer/tablet/phone, you'll have everything you need at your fingertips so that you can easily share the latest information with anyone who requires it.

While you may be tempted to organize this material electronically, there are pitfalls with this strategy. First, you may be caring for your LO for a long time, and technology breaks and changes, which means that you will be moving information from one device to another and possibly losing it. The cloud you're storing scanned documents in can be hacked. You may show up for a doctor appointment only to find that you can't connect to their Wi-Fi. My advice: stick with a low-tech binder, because you're going to need a paper backup anyway.

In 2014, the Electronic Medical Records (EMR) Mandate was passed, which requires all healthcare providers to convert their handwritten medical charts to a digital format. This means that your LO's charts can be accessed and downloaded and easily added to your binder. You and your LO will have to set up an account on each medical provider's patient portal if they are not affiliated with the same hospital or system. Make sure you write down the username and password.

Your binder should be divided into sections for each of their specialists, with lists of their medications, appointments, and the notes you take after each office visit. Then, when you see your LO's primary care provider, you can make sure that they are aware of what the specialists are prescribing and testing.

THE CAREGIVER'S ENEMY: STRESS

The only effective caregiver is a healthy caregiver, and I mean sound in body, mind, and spirit. The number one mistake I see caregivers make is taking on too much and not taking care of themselves. The consequences are real. Chronic stress shrinks a part of the brain called the *hippocampus*, and when that happens, your attention span, perception, long-term memory, learning, and word-finding diminishes. That sounds like the makings of dementia to me.

Remember my friend Ernest from the last chapter? I believe that his stress level from taking care of his mother increased his own risk for developing dementia. Now that he has the diagnosis as well, his wife, Dominque, doesn't want the same thing to happen to her, which is why her daughter, Kelsey, is helping to relieve the load.

Dominique is absolutely doing the right thing for herself and her husband, because two caregivers will be able to support each other and ultimately deliver better care. If you make sure to have some downtime every day, and you have identified people to turn to when you need a break, you will be setting yourself up for success.

Rest assured, this book will help you get you through the biggest hurdles. I'm not saying that every day is going to be fun. There will be times when you get angry. There will be times when caregiving is frustrating. There will be times when you feel guilty. You're entitled to experience a full range of emotions. You're also entitled to take a break. On the days when you're really struggling, you are entitled to seek help from someone else. That's why the team approach is critical. If you set up your teams now, you will avoid chronic caregiver stress.

CREATING THE IDEAL TEAMS

The best caregivers build multiple teams of people they can turn to for support. And they use these teams and *let them help*, instead of taking on all the responsibility themselves. One of the most frequent mistakes caregivers make is saying that they want to delegate responsibilities but not actually doing so. They may be afraid that others will judge their abilities as a caregiver, or that no one else will be as good a caregiver as they are. In order to continue having a balanced life, you are going to have to delegate and put in processes that others can follow.

Since 2008, *60 Minutes* has been following a married couple, Mike and Carol Daly, in a recurring segment called "For Better or Worse." That year, Carol was diagnosed with AD,[1] and she and Mike made a pact that he would be her only caregiver until the end of her life. Dr. Jon LaPook interviews the couple every year to chronicle her cognitive decline. What always stood out for me is how poorly Mike has done over the past decade-plus: he developed high blood pressure, gained an enormous amount of weight, and is facing severe depression. In 2018, Mike said on the show, "I should have never kept that pact. It was too much." Ultimately, he was forced to put his wife in a nursing home, for which he feels enormous guilt. While we can't judge the choices made by others under impossible circumstances, I can't help but wonder: had he taken a team approach from the beginning, could he have kept Carol at home?

If you're up to the task of being the caregiver, your team will handle some of the details that you can't provide, that you don't want to provide, or that you will need help providing. Then you will develop what I call a *Family Care Plan* to identify exactly when team members should regularly come to your aid.

There are two teams you need to fill: your LO's family and friends who pitch in on a regular basis, and the professionals and other people who will make your life easier.

Track Your Teams in Your Binder

Record the names of people who you think will be best suited to fill each role for the two teams. As your LO progresses through the disease, these names will likely change. Think about what type of help you need now, and how that may shift as your responsibilities grow. You'll also be able to adjust your teams as the members of your support system get comfortable with their roles. Hopefully, they will be able to take on additional responsibilities as caregiving becomes more challenging.

TEAM #1: FAMILY AND FRIENDS

Once you decide to take on the role of the primary caregiver, the next step is to see who in the family or your friend group will play supporting roles. Every person, from grandchildren up, can provide some aspect of caregiving. The key is to set up a schedule in your Family Care Plan, so that everyone knows when and how they are expected to pitch in (see sample Family Care Plans at the end of the chapter).

There are loads of ways someone else can lend a hand, even if it's as simple as taking your LO for a walk. If you have family members who live far away, they could provide coverage for a week or two, twice a year. They can take on managing your LO's finances and bills and schedule weekly calls or video chats with your LO so that you can prepare meals. Someone else can put together a simple photo album or poster that highlights the people your LO will be seeing frequently. Label each photograph with the person's name and how they fit into your LO's life. It can also be a storytelling tool: use it to keep your LO in the loop of what's happening within the family by pointing to their picture as you share the latest news and gossip.

Friends or family who live close by can help you with these aspects of caregiving, regardless of what stage your LO is in:

- Housekeeping
- Meal prep/cooking
- Grocery shopping (in person or coordinating online shopping)
- Covering for you for an hour or two every day so that you can take a break
- Friendly visiting: coming over to be with your LO to maintain socialization skills
- Taking your LO shopping, to the supermarket, or to a movie (until they can no longer do the activity without getting agitated)

Keep Everyone in the Loop

If you have an extended family or a large circle of friends, talk about roles and responsibilities early on. Just because you are taking on this role doesn't mean that you have to go it alone. It also doesn't mean that your parent loves you more. Sometimes all it means is that you live closer or have more time or resources to devote right now.

It will be your responsibility to keep Team #1 in the loop. For example, when you notice major shifts in behaviors, or if a doctor tells you that your LO is moving from the mild to the moderate stages, everyone in the family needs to be updated. Weekly conference calls or Zoom meetings provide everyone with the most current information; they also are a forum so that you can get their input, tips, and ideas.

TEAM #2: MY "OUTSIDE THE FAMILY" DREAM TEAM

I have put together the players for this second team based on my work at dementia care facilities, where the team approach is the only model of care. Every two weeks or so, there is a team meeting for each resident. Family members and the resident themselves are encouraged to participate. The team discusses the resident's care plan for the next two weeks and which members of the team will be required each day.

You can re-create the same type of team approach for your home, and your job is to manage everybody on this team. The team members will also change based on the needs of your LO and what stage they are in. However, it's a good idea to identify who will fill these roles before they are even needed and find out if you need a referral from your LO's primary physician to see them. Identify every service that your LO is entitled to as part of their Medicare, Medicaid, or health insurance plans. Search the internet for their LO's local Department of Aging; many communities provide services either through their town or nonprofits that you may be able to receive.

Your professional support team will include:

Primary care physician (PCP): This person sits at the hub of your LO's medical wheel and coordinates all specialist care and medications. The PCP needs to specialize in treating dementia/AD patients. Look for someone who is affiliated with the local hospital and part of an established geriatric practice—a group that specializes in treating the elderly, even if your LO is not yet elderly (if they have early-onset dementia/AD), and has relationships with other geriatric specialists. This way, they can make recommendations for specialists that are within the same insurance plan and hospital system. They should be able to talk to your LO with respect, keeping in mind their cognitive abilities. Remember, you get to pick the right doctor: some physicians, even those who specialize in geriatrics, cannot simplify their language enough to make someone with dementia/AD feel comfortable.

Neurologist: This is a doctor who specializes in brain function and health. Choose one whose practice is linked to your PCP and who focuses on dementia symptoms and disease progression. The neurologist is going to do a number of cognitive screening tests in order to confirm the diagnosis.

Medical specialists: Depending on your LO's preexisting health issues, they may need to be seen regularly by other doctors. In fact, this is quite likely, because dementia does not occur in a vacuum. Often patients have other health issues as well; for example, they may need an endocrinologist to treat diabetes or a podiatrist to deal with their feet. Make sure all of the specialists are in the same hospital system and insurance plan. Your PCP will be able to tell you what other health conditions need to be monitored.

Audiologist/ear, nose, and throat (ENT) specialist: A hearing test is not part of the typical annual physical. Yet your LO's hearing needs to be assessed every year because poor hearing can exacerbate dementia symptoms. Once your LO has an ENT in place, the ENT can update the PCP with your LO's test results.

Occupational therapist (OT): OTs enhance independence by addressing the ADLs that your LO may be struggling with. Depending on your LO's health insurance, OT services may require a referral from their PCP. You can also find an OT and pay for their services yourself. They are most useful to seek out in the early and moderate stages.

Physical therapist (PT): PTs recognize and correct physical behaviors and symptoms, such as walking with a limp or developing pain in the neck or shoulders resulting from constantly looking at the floor. Depending on your LO's health insurance, PT services may require a referral from their PCP. You can also find one and pay for their services yourself if you notice that your LO is in pain or holding an unusual posture. PTs are most often used in the early and moderate stages.

Nutritionist/dietitian: If your LO shows a marked increase or decrease in weight, you will want to bring in a food specialist who can tweak their diet as needed. A nutritionist can also help your LO choose healthy foods they will enjoy to replace bad eating habits. Some insurance policies will cover the cost of a nutritionist. These professionals can be called in at any stage.

Social worker: A social worker is a private hire. They will evaluate your LO and their family to see what social services they may benefit from and are entitled to from local and federal government. In my experience, you have to ask the social worker to recommend services: they are not always forthcoming. Don't be shy if you find that you need more help. Ask, *"I need help. What services am I entitled to?"* A clinical social worker is covered by Medicare and Medicaid: they provide mental health therapy for your LO and may work with you and the rest of your family to improve family dynamics. You can request a social worker at any stage; check your LO's insurance and contact your local hospital for references. However, any time your LO is in the hospital, always request a meeting with the social worker while they are admitted. The social worker will provide information for additional services for when your LO is back at home.

Case manager: This person helps families resolve issues regarding treatments and services, and they flag medical problems for insurance companies. Your LO's insurance company, including Medicare (and the supplemental insurances) and Medicaid, will send a case manager to the home every six months to check on your LO's overall health, making sure that they are keeping up with doctor appointments and medications. This case manager may be a social worker or a professional nurse. You can hire a case manager at any stage.

Geriatric care manager: This person is a private hire. They are typically a former nurse or social worker and are certified to help you find resources and services for your LO. They navigate government and nonprofit systems and can act as an advocate for your LO to receive the services they are entitled to. A geriatric case manager can be used at any stage; you can find one through the community's social service agency or local hospital.

Attorney: An attorney puts together the documents to codify your LO's wishes and their permission for you to make medical decisions on their behalf. They explain the benefits that your state or other organizations offer and how to allocate their assets to take advantage of them. For instance, if your LO is a veteran or a member of a nonprofit organization like the Masons, they may be entitled to eldercare at significantly reduced costs.

Supplemental care provider: This role is filled by Medicaid. If your LO is entitled to this service, a person will come for a set of hours, paid for by the state, to assist you with home care. There are specific chores that a supplemental care provider is allowed to do, including helping you fix meals, clean the home, and watch your LO. As the primary caregiver, you manage this person. This role can also be filled by a family member, through your LO's long-term health insurance, or through a private agency where you will pay for their services. A supplemental care person can be called in at any stage.

Volunteers from local nonprofit agencies: There may be nonprofits in your LO's community that organize volunteers to help with various tasks. They may do grocery shopping, light housekeeping, home repair, or friendly visiting. Find out which local nonprofits can help get you a break for at least an hour.

Housekeeper/meal provider/grocery shopper/finance manager: Make sure that these aspects of managing the household are covered because your LO will not be able to perform them once they enter the moderate stages. These are all jobs performed by members of Team #1 to lighten your load.

Adult daycare and/or community centers: These agencies provide activities for socialization outside the home. During the early stages, your LO can be dropped off for a set window of time each day or certain days during the week. In the later stages, you may have to accompany them, at which point you will have to determine if it is worthwhile.

Transportation services: Many towns offer transportation for doctor visits and grocery shopping, or to adult daycare facilities. Check your local government's website to see what's available.

End-of-life doula or palliative care/hospice nurse: An end-of-life doula offers a spiritual focus on bereavement as well as technical expertise on the medical aspects of hospice care. Hospice care is ordered by your LO's PCP, and it doesn't have to coincide with end of life: it can also be ordered for palliative care—relieving pain and troubling symptoms that affect quality of life—at any of the earlier stages. Hospice care is funded by the federal government, but it's managed by each state, and each state has its own rules and regulations. Learn what your state provides so that you can take advantage of this critical service.

> **Take Your LO into Account When Planning Team #2**
>
> Your LO may require additional team members, and I believe "the more, the merrier." For instance, if your LO is a churchgoer, they may want to add their minister and church friends as part of their team. Some ministers do home visits well before end of life. They can also participate in Zoom calls to break up the day.
>
> This is one area where being an open-minded caregiver pays off. Sometimes adding people to the network can provide a new perspective on your LO's health status, especially if you slip into denial or become overprotective. These people knew your LO well before their illness, in a totally different way than you may have experienced them. They may have participated in an ongoing card game or book club, or they may have met for coffee at a specific spot. Listen to what they have to say with an open heart and adjust your care accordingly.

INVESTIGATE PACE

If putting Team #2 together seems like a daunting task, the U.S. government offers a program that makes it easier. The Program of All-Inclusive Care for the Elderly (PACE) is literally re-creating nursing home care delivered right in your LO's own home. Sound familiar?

PACE provides the following benefits and, depending what state your LO lives in, these benefits are covered by either Medicaid, Medicare, or both:

- Adult daycare
- Dentistry
- Emergency services

- End-of-life care
- Home care
- Hospital care
- Laboratory/X-ray services
- Meals
- Medical specialty services
- Nutritional counseling
- Occupational therapy
- Physical therapy
- Prescription drugs
- Primary care (including doctor and nursing services)
- Recreational therapy
- Social services
- Social work counseling
- Transportation

To participate, your LO must be at least 55 years old and qualify for nursing home care based on the ADL list in Chapter 1. If they qualify, you have to do a bit of research. PACE is a national initiative that individual states manage through private care companies. For example, there are only six places in all of New York State that participate. So while it may be in your state, it may not be offered in your community. PACE providers are typically a nonprofit private or public entity that already provides healthcare services.

Once your LO is enrolled in PACE, you have to use the services they provide: you can't choose in an "à la carte" fashion your team members versus theirs. PACE providers receive monthly Medicare and/or Medicaid payments for each enrollee depending on the state they are operating in. If your LO doesn't qualify for Medicaid, you pay monthly premiums equal to what Medicaid would charge without additional deductibles, coinsurance, or any other cost sharing.

PACE is a realistic option if your LO is on the younger spectrum of dementia/AD and you want or need to continue working. It provides all of the care your LO will need and gives you peace of mind that they are being well taken care of, in their own home, while you are at your job. Best of all, you can end the program at any time if it doesn't meet your expectations.

GET YOUR LO'S PAPERWORK IN ORDER

As an LPN and an MBA, I understand the ideal intersection of financial planning and healthcare, and it's always at the beginning of the process. Find an eldercare attorney to help you review your LO's finances and existing health insurance as soon as possible, so that you

---

Your LO Deserves All the Services They Are Entitled To

If your family has always been self-reliant, it may be hard to accept the team approach. You may not see the value of having strangers come into your home to clean, or the need to draw on public services. However, I advise you to quickly get past your pride and see what programs and services are available. Not only is your LO likely to get better care, but you will receive much-needed support, too.

Government services aren't a handout: your LO has been paying for these services all along through their taxes. Now it's their turn to collect. Think of these programs like a car insurance policy: you make a payment every month, and when you have an accident, your insurance covers your claim.

---

know what your options are. Your LO may be able to afford more than you know, including private nursing (full-time or part-time, or even hourly). Or their health or long-term insurance may provide benefits that make caregiving easier.

Your LO should also have a plan for their end of life that they develop with their eldercare attorney. This plan needs to be formulated while they can still make decisions about the hard questions: if they wait until they are no longer competent, many of these documents are not legally binding. Don't be surprised if your LO has definitive ideas of what their end of life should look like: according to a 2018 *New York Times* article, 90 percent of people who make these decisions specifically limit end-of-life care to "comfort only" and not the additional heroic measures that can ensure "longevity."[2] That means you may have to come around to your LO's wishes and accept them for what they are.

While some of the recommended documents can be downloaded from the Internet, it's best to have a professional look all of them over. Then figure out a place where you are going to keep them and let everyone else in the family know. My friend Pamela Macon works with families and individuals facing end-of-life decisions by organizing their necessary paperwork. She explained to me that there is dignity in having one's health trajectory align with their expressed wishes. Too many families do not make plans, or don't know how to generate or where to store paperwork. In fact, most people with dementia/AD do not have an end-of-life plan in place.[3] This is a critical mistake that is easily fixed. The cost of preparing the necessary paperwork is far less than the drama that will result if you don't have it in order.

These documents are referred to as *advance directives*. Many will influence each other: for example, you need both a healthcare proxy *and* a living will; otherwise, decisions are left in the hands of the caregiver and may not reflect what their LO really wants.

The key legal and medical documents to have on hand when you start caregiving are the following:

Living will: a formalization of your LO's wishes for medical treatment, including artificial life support. If they do not want to be revived in the hospital or at home, the living will needs to contain a clause referred to as a DNR (do not resuscitate).

Standard will: a formal declaration of your LO's wishes regarding the disposal of property and savings after death.

Power of attorney: a formal document that gives an individual—who should be the primary caregiver but can also be another friend or family member—the ability to make financial decisions on behalf of the LO when they are incapable of doing so. If your LO assigns both financial and healthcare decisions to one person, the formal name for this document is a *durable power of attorney for healthcare*. The informal name is a *healthcare proxy*.

HIPAA release form: The Health Insurance Portability and Accountability Act of 1996 (HIPAA) is a federal law that protects sensitive patient health information from being disclosed without a patient's consent. A HIPAA release allows your LO to authorize their health providers to disclose their health information to you, or anyone of their choosing. You will need this authorization in order to have frank conversations with your LO's doctors and be part of the decision-making process.

Once you have these documents, keep a copy of each in your binder. Your LO should keep a copy with their attorney, in a safe location in the home, or in a safe-deposit box at their local bank.

Collecting Social Security and Splitting Assets

If you are caring for a spouse and would like them to be considered for Medicaid or additional services your state provides, consider formally separating your finances and assets. By doing so, you are not legally bound to the financial responsibilities of their care, and they may be entitled to more aid.

Your LO may also qualify for additional government subsidies. The Social Security Administration includes all of the following among the list of conditions under its Compassionate Allowances (CAL) initiative, giving your LO earlier access to Social Security Disability Insurance and Supplemental Security Income:

- Early-onset Alzheimer's disease
- Adult-onset Huntington disease
- Creutzfeldt-Jakob disease (CJD)
- Frontotemporal dementia (FTD)
- Lewy body dementia
- Mixed dementia

BUILDING A FAMILY CARE PLAN

A Family Care Plan is the backbone of caregiving. I've based this idea on the care plan that professional nurses use to provide and guide their daily care. Nurses use it to make sure that they are implementing a team approach and that team members have access to meet their client's medical and personal needs. By doing so, nurses ensure that the team is fully integrated, which means that the burden of care is not solely on their shoulders and they do not fall victim to caregiver stress.

Your Family Care Plan should be set for a week or two at a time and then broken down into smaller increments. It can be as detailed as you want, including tasks such as daily grooming, paying the bills, and housekeeping. Most important, every day, you're going to build in a break for yourself.

Keep in mind that dementia/AD are conditions that are guaranteed to change. You will modify your Family Care Plan every time your LO shows some form of decline: as they lose the ability to participate in certain activities, or if more team members need to come in to provide specific new services.

SAMPLE FAMILY CARE PLAN FOR EARLY/MILD STAGES

If you are lucky enough to have your LO properly diagnosed in Stage 1, 2, or 3, they may very well be able to continue to live by themselves and maintain much of their independence. As the primary caregiver, you must take the time to observe them carefully and note any changes as they come up. You may help your LO accomplish their *instrumental activities of daily living* (IADLs) like household chores, grocery shopping, meal prep/cooking, managing finances, and arranging doctor appointments. Many of these tasks can be completed in your own home, away from your LO. That's why this early-stages Family Care Plan will be less about constant monitoring and more about checking in to make sure that your LO is safe and able to continue to perform their ADLs covered in Chapter 1.

In these early stages your Family Care Plan should begin to schedule informal, friendly visits from your Team #1 members, as well as the times when you will accompany your LO on doctor appointments. As the disease progresses, incorporate more support into the Family

Care Plan. For example, add a housekeeper or a grocery shopper if your LO is no longer up to the task and you don't have the time.

Even in the early stages your LO may benefit from keeping a loose schedule. This will help them complete tasks without getting overwhelmed, especially if they are still working. I always recommend to my families that they schedule all doctor appointments on the same day of the week. It's easier for you to remember and block out your own schedule, as you will be attending them. It is also easier for your LO because it becomes part of their routine. Best of all, your LO may be able to slow the progression of the disease in the early stages by using a schedule and relying on others for support. These tools will keep them calmer throughout the day when they know that someone is there to help out if needed.

Here's a typical weekly schedule for the early/mild stages, assuming that your LO is living independently and cooks for themselves. Invite your LO to help you make a schedule that works for them. Make sure to include specific times each day when they will have visitors or support people. Not only will these people help them retain their autonomy, they will provide much-needed company, as loneliness contributes to dementia decline.

Sunday	Church/lunch visit with friends Clean home with Team #1 or #2 member Exercise: at least a half-hour walk
Monday	Grocery shopping or online ordering alone or with primary caregiver Exercise: at least a half-hour walk
Tuesday	Team #2 doctor appointments Exercise: at least a half-hour walk Visit with Team #1 member
Wednesday	Lunch/dinner with primary caregiver Exercise: at least a half-hour walk

Thursday	Pay bills Exercise: at least a half-hour walk Team #1 member checks in
Friday	Exercise: at least a half-hour walk Movie night
Saturday	Personal grooming: hair/nails Exercise: at least a half-hour walk Dinner with friends/family

SAMPLE FAMILY CARE PLAN FOR MODERATE STAGES

By the end of Stage 3, and certainly at the beginning of Stage 4, your LO requires 24-hour supervision. While you likely won't assist with toileting yet, your LO is no longer safe at home alone. This is most often the stage where the family is forced to snap out of denial as a result of some sort of accident: a fender bender, a fall getting in or out of the shower, or a kitchen incident. The principal mistake caregivers make at this point is believing that their LO only needs supervision during the day. Besides the risk of a fall in the middle of the night, this is when people with dementia/AD start to wander or hallucinate, which means that they need to be supervised day and night.

At the same time, they may start feeling uncomfortable around a wide assortment of people. In order for you to take a break, slot one team member into the Family Care Plan per day, and be as consistent as possible. With family, that may mean that Cousin Lucy commits to Tuesdays at 4:00 p.m., and Uncle Larry comes over Saturday afternoons for lunch.

The moderate-stage Family Care Plan shows when you and your LO need to leave the house and when your support team members come over. This is an ideal time to introduce adult daycare at least a few times a week, which will provide you with a long window of free time. Adult daycare is not a substitute for live-in care: you still need to be with your LO when they get up in the morning to get them ready to go, provide breakfast, and potentially pack a lunch. As the disease progresses, your LO may not be able to attend daycare without you, and at that point you will have to evaluate whether it's worth the effort to get them out of the house.

The Family Care Plan can also schedule team members for weekly chores, like housekeeping. If you find someone outside the family who can help out on a regular basis, they can also develop a relationship with your LO. As they develop their trust, they may be able to monitor your LO while they clean, and you can get a break. My aunt had a housekeeper, Betsy, come for 4 hours every Monday morning. It only took Betsy an hour and a half to clean the house, and then she spent the rest of her time visiting with my aunt. They went for walks, or folded the clothes, or prepared lunch together. Best of all, we were introduced to Betsy through a local nonprofit, which had a grant to pay housekeepers. That meant that she came at no cost to help my aunt, and my cousin could count on that window every Monday to take a long break.

Keep in mind, though, that anyone who is remotely connected to a health-related service—the occupational therapist, the physical therapist, the social worker, or the case manager—will require you to stick around for the appointment. You should not rely on secondhand information about your LO's status from either the provider or your LO.

Continue to schedule all doctor appointments on the same day, but now you need to make the window for appointments smaller, as your LO gets tired more easily. For instance, stick with Tuesdays as the medical day, but schedule all of the appointments between 10:00 a.m. and 1:00 p.m.

The following is a sample Family Care Plan for a moderate-stage Sunday. Coverage can be provided by the same person at different times, or one person for one time during the day; remember, you don't want lots of different people coming in and out of the home, which will cause confusion for your LO.

Sunday Time	Schedule for Loved One (LO)	Opportunities for Caregiver Free Time
8:00 a.m.	Morning ADLs: bathing, grooming, dressing	
9:00 a.m.	Prepare breakfast, eat breakfast, clean up after breakfast	
10:00 a.m.	Church service (online or in person), including travel time	Caregiver free time, if you have coverage
11:00 a.m.		
12:00 p.m.	Prepare lunch, eat lunch, clean up after lunch	
1:00 p.m.	Exercise for caregiver and LO	
2:00 p.m.	Family/friends visit	Caregiver free time
3:00 p.m.		
4:00 p.m.	Activity: Prepare dinner and set table	
5:00 p.m.	Eat dinner, clean up after dinner	
6:00 p.m.	Activity (see Chapter 6)	Caregiver free time, if you have coverage
7:00 p.m.	Television/reading	Caregiver free time
8:00 p.m.	Prepare for bed, bedtime snack	
9:00 p.m.	Bedtime	Caregiver free time once the LO is asleep

Other typical free time windows during a moderate-stage week:

- Adult daycare: half or full day
- Volunteer/supplemental care person: 2 hours or a half day
- Housekeeper: 2 hours or a half day if they are a trusted resource to keep an eye on your LO *and* you speak the same language

SAMPLE FAMILY CARE PLAN FOR LATE STAGES

Stage 6 marks the beginning of the late or severe stage. The moderate and severe Family Care Plans are similar, but the time frame for activities will be shorter. As your LO progresses through the disease, they may only be able to do two activities a day instead of three. They may no longer be able to go to adult daycare. They may need more than one nap during the day. The severe plan also includes toileting, first as a reminder, and later as a chore.

As your LO progresses further into the severe stages, there are fewer opportunities to get them out of the house. The case manager becomes a more prominent team member, and your LO can receive other services from Medicare, Medicaid, and their insurance company.

You will still want someone to come every day to give you a break, and members of Team #1 are your likely resources. Unlike the moderate stages, at this point your LO is not as stressed by having different people come in over the course of the day, because they aren't as likely to be as agitated by strangers (and at that point, most people are "strangers" to them), so a variety of family members can help you out on the same day.

The following is a sample Family Care Plan for a severe-stage Monday. Coverage can be provided by the same person at different times, or different people at different times.

Monday Time	Schedule for Loved One (LO)	Opportunities for Caregiver Free Time
8:00 a.m.	Morning ADLs: bathing, grooming, dressing	
9:00 a.m.	Prepare breakfast, eat breakfast, clean up after breakfast	

Monday Time	Schedule for Loved One (LO)	Opportunities for Caregiver Free Time
9:45 a.m.	Toileting (and the transition to addressing incontinence—see Chapter 5)	
10:00 a.m.	Craft activity (see Chapter 6)	
10:45 a.m.	Snack	
11:00 a.m.	OT/exercise for LO only	
11:45 a.m.	Toileting	
12:00 p.m.	Prepare lunch, eat lunch, clean up after lunch	
1:00 p.m.	Television/reading/rest time	Caregiver free time, if you have coverage
1:45 p.m.	Toileting	
2:00 p.m.	Family/friends visit/volunteer	Caregiver free time
3:00 p.m.		
3:45 p.m.	Toileting	
4:00 p.m.	Rest time for LO: caregiver preps dinner	
5:00 p.m.	Eat dinner, clean up after dinner	
5:45 p.m.	Toileting	
6:00 p.m.	Activity with team member	Caregiver free time
7:00 p.m.	Prepare for bed, bedtime snack, toileting	
8:00 p.m.	Bedtime	Caregiver free time once the LO is asleep

Other typical team member visits for a severe-stage week:

- OT/PT/social worker/case manager/geriatric care manager/ hospice doctor or nurse
- Volunteer/supplemental care person: 2 hours or a half day
- Housekeeper: 2 hours or a half day if they are a trusted resource to keep an eye on your LO *and* you speak the same language

Stage 7, or end of life, means that your LO is likely to be bedridden. They are not walking or feeding themselves. While you may not need a detailed Family Care Plan, you still need to schedule in free time for yourself (a rough plan is included in Chapter 10). Caregiving at this stage is literally a hands-on affair, which makes it both physically and mentally draining. Ideally, you should be rotating daily caregiving with other members of your team, including family and hospice providers.

While it may seem like it is a long way off, identify now who you will be able to count on later. Ask family members who are physically fit if they will be able to alternate days or follow a day/night shift schedule. Spiritual leaders and end-of-life doulas offer tremendous support to both you and your LO during these final weeks.

THE LOVE AND JOY OF CAREGIVING

Building teams is one of the best ways to prevent caregiver burnout. Yet there will still be days that can best be described as challenging. That doesn't mean that on those same days, you won't be happy. Happiness comes from within, and no one and nothing else can take that away. Most of all, happiness comes from living a life of purpose. And what's more purposeful than caregiving?

Happiness also comes from the act of loving another, and to me, caregiving is the ultimate act of love. When you combine love with the happiness of purpose, you will be able to get through even the toughest days with grace. In the next chapters, we'll keep the focus on you and provide real tools to help you make sense of the most challenging days.

CHAPTER 3

Self-Care Strategies:
Taking Care of the Caregiver

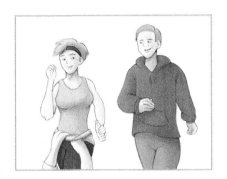

Caregiving requires both physical and mental stamina, so it's best to prepare for the entire journey. And the best way to prepare yourself is to take care of yourself. Far too often, caregivers are physically taxed, emotionally burdened, isolated, and in poor health. Yet professional caregivers like me are in better shape than the typical family member who is caring for a loved one. The reason is simple: I make time for me every single day, even when I'm hired for providing 24/7 care. I've found that when caregivers take care of themselves, they are better prepared to go the distance, all the while providing excellent care for their LO. Best of all, when you're mentally and physically healthy, you will be able to relax and enjoy the new relationship between you and your LO.

Let's talk through how I take care of myself even when I'm taking care of a patient. As you'll see, these suggestions can easily be adjusted to match the caregiving needs of your LO.

USE YOUR FAMILY CARE PLAN

I can't stress enough how critical it is to use the Family Care Plan to map out your day, as well as your LO's. Identify and then schedule specific times when your team members should come over and give you a break. Then chart out what you need to accomplish on these breaks. Think about when you will run errands or see your own friends. Again, the earlier you set up the expectation that others should help you—and then really allow them to help—the better.

When you are with your LO, your free time will always be determined by their mental and physical abilities: what stage of the disease they are in and their safety. This is another reason why every Family Care Plan is a short-term strategy: when it comes to dementia/AD, your LO's abilities may decline quickly and drastically. For example, if your LO is in the beginning of Stage 3, you may be able to exercise in another room while they are watching television. By the end of the same stage, your LO may wander out of the home while you're working out, so your days of exercising without keeping an eye on them are over.

Use your Family Care Plan to schedule in self-care. In the early stages, you and your LO can do many of these activities together, like meditate, watch a movie, listen to music, or exercise. In the moderate and later stages, these same activities will more often be split: you'll read aloud to your LO a book that is appropriate for their cognitive level, and then later, after you put them to bed, you'll be able to focus on one you enjoy.

Plan a Monthly Spa Day

You deserve one full day every month that is completely dedicated to self-care, so work it into your Family Care Plan from the start. Pick a weekday as opposed to a weekend so that you can get to your own doctor appointments, the hair salon, and so on. Then make sure you have coverage from a team member, or two who can split the day. Or use an adult daycare center if your LO can attend on their own.

Plan in advance what you want to accomplish and schedule appointments ahead of time. Take extra care of your feet because they are supporting your whole body. A massage can help you release the tension you are carrying. Not only does a good haircut or manicure make it easier for you to get up and get going in the morning, but we all feel better when we know we are looking our best. Exercise at a gym, see your doctor or therapist, or just have lunch with a friend: it's your day. If you're on a tight budget, look for a Groupon for discount services, or ask a friend to swap services: you do their nails, and they will do yours.

This time off will really feel like a vacation, even though you aren't going far away. Knowing that your LO is in good hands and you are completely off duty will give you the opportunity to step out of your day-to-day, relax, and rejuvenate. You'll return to your LO with a clear head so that you can come up with creative solutions to new problems as they arise.

MAKE TIME TO EAT HEALTHFULLY

I took this tip from the Millennial playbook because these hard workers have it right: meal prep saves time and lowers stress. Meal prep means preparing whole meals, or certain ingredients, like vegetables, ahead of time. It guarantees that your favorite meals are ready to eat and stored in portions so that you don't overindulge. You can block out an afternoon on your Family Care Plan for prepping dinners for the next five days. Or take an hour to prep vegetables, grains such as rice, or cooked meats so you can speed up the cooking process later in the week. Once meal prep is in your Family Care Plan, all you'll need is lots of meal-sized containers for storage.

Even easier if you can afford them are meal delivery services that provide nutritious frozen meals, or fresh ingredients already prepped for cooking. You can cross off cooking from your to-do list, and you gain back the time it takes to shop for and prepare fresh meals. What's more, flash-frozen foods stay fresh for a long time without losing quality. It's worth exploring these services to have a few weeks' worth of frozen meals on hand for those days when you need extra help. There are services that cater to specialized diets, like vegan or paleo, and the following are good choices for maintaining a well-balanced, healthy diet. Many can also be personalized for specific dietary needs:

- Fresh foods prepped with recipes: Blue Apron, Green Chef, HelloFresh
- Freshly prepared frozen meals: Freshly, Magic Kitchen, Balance by BistroMD

Your diet should consist of lean proteins—from animal sources, dairy, or beans—along with colorful fruits and vegetables and healthy fats, like olive oil, yogurt, or avocado. Luckily, these are many of the same choices you'll be making for your LO, which makes meal prep and sticking to the right diet easier. I've also found that the best approach is to balance each meal, so if you have the occasional fast food, it won't throw off your entire day. Lastly, you're going to need to drink lots of water. Caregiving can be physically taxing, and staying hydrated is one of the best ways to keep your energy levels high. Keep healthy snacks handy for when you need a quick shot of energy. I don't need to tell you that it's easy to reach for a donut instead of an apple when you're tired, but I will tell you that I haven't met too many caregivers who have lost weight. So be gentle on yourself; reward yourself with your favorite treat every once in a while, but more often, take care of yourself by sticking to a healthy diet. It takes a lot of hard work to undo bad eating habits. And if you can't shake them, they'll have serious consequences for your health.

Lastly, sit down for meals. If there is one thing your LO has plenty of, it's time. You don't need to eat over the kitchen sink or scarf down a sandwich. Sit down, enjoy the meal you've prepared, and appreciate their company.

EXERCISE FOR 30 MINUTES EVERY DAY

Exercise not only strengthens muscles and increases endurance, it decreases stress and improves brain function, so if you want to be at your best, you need to exercise for at least 30 minutes every day. Again, start with your Family Care Plan. Look at your schedule and see how are you going to fit in a workout. In the early stages you will be able to leave your LO for an hour, and you should take advantage of that time and start developing an exercise habit. During the moderate and severe stages, you will not be able to leave your LO alone, so you will have to get a little more creative. Can you work out when a team member is covering for you, or when your LO takes a nap?

I group exercise into two categories: stress relief and physical fitness. The best exercises cross over and address both of these categories at the same time. However, sometimes you just need a little stress relief: that's when restorative yoga or tai chi comes in handy. You can find routines that match your time availability on the Internet.

GET YOURSELF FIT WITH NIK

If you already have an exercise routine, keep going. If you don't, now is a great time to start. My friend Nikki Kimbrough is one of the top fitness experts in the United States. She developed the following physical fitness program just for you, to address the specific needs of caregivers. You can do this 30-minute cardio/strength training routine at home, without any equipment, to clear your head and keep your whole body strong.

Nikki breaks down this routine into sections or circuits that are meant to be completed sequentially. You can also break it up over the course of the day, although make sure to do the warm-up and cooldown every time. The total time for each section is a goal: if you haven't exercised in a while, it may take you a little longer. That's fine; it's never too late to get into shape. As you get stronger and more fit, you can double the entire workout in the same amount of time.

The descriptions for each move are given after the workouts that follow. There are also "options" to make the workout a bit easier. If you want to follow along as Nikki goes through the routine, check out www.getfitwithnik.com/caregiving-with-love-joy.

WARM-UP
- Inhale/Exhale (2x)
- Hip Circles (Left and Right)

- Neck Rolls
- Shoulder Rolls
- Big Arm Circles
- Flexion/Extension
- Reach and Pull
- Standing Hamstring Stretch (Left and Right)
- Standing Quad Stretch
- Inhale/Exhale (2x)

CIRCUIT 1: CARDIO
- Jog in Place—10 Seconds
- Jumping Jacks—45 Seconds (Option: Side-to-Side Jacks)
- Jump Rope—45 Seconds (Option: Bounce in Place of Jump)
- Heel-Toe—45 Seconds (Option: Heel-Toe Bounce Step)
- Squat to Press—45 Seconds

CIRCUIT 2: STRENGTH
- Romanian Deadlift to Row—45 Seconds
- Triceps Kickbacks to Upward Pulse—45 Seconds
- Horizontal Wood Chop Left—45 Seconds
- Horizontal Wood Chop Right—45 Seconds

CIRCUIT 3: CARDIO
- Heel-Toe (Single, Single, Double)—45 Seconds (Option: Bounce)
- Squat to Kick—45 Seconds
- Inchworm Push-Ups—45 Seconds (Option: Inchworm to Knee Push-Ups)
- Supermans—45 Seconds
- Crunches—45 Seconds

CIRCUIT 4: STRENGTH
- Romanian Deadlift to Fly—45 Seconds
- Alt Reverse Lunge to Bicep Curls—45 Seconds
- Diagonal Wood Chop Left—45 Seconds
- Diagonal Wood Chop Right—45 Seconds

CIRCUIT 5: CARDIO
- Heel-Toe (Low to High)—45 Seconds (Option: Heel-Toe Bounce)
- Squats (Out/Out/In/In Pulse)—45 Seconds
- Mountain Climbers—45 Seconds (Option: add a chair)
- Bicycle Crunches—45 Seconds
- Push-Ups—45 Seconds (Option: Push-Ups on Knees)

COOL-DOWN
- Bring Both Knees into Chest and Rock Side to Side
- Flagpole Stretch (Right)
- Cross-over-Spine Stretch (Right)
- Floor Quad Stretch (Right)
- Flagpole Stretch (Left)
- Cross-over-Spine Stretch (Left)
- Floor Quad Stretch (Left)
- Upward Dog
- Child's Pose
- Shoulder Stretch
- Roll Up to Shoulder Rolls
- Extension/Flexion
- Inhale/Exhale

Exercise Descriptions/Instructions

WARM-UP

HIP CIRCLES (LEFT AND RIGHT)

- Stand straight with your feet a little wider than shoulder width apart. Bend your knees slightly and place your hands on your hips.
- Slowly rotate your hips, making big circles.
- Complete a set in one direction and then switch to the opposite direction.

NECK ROLLS

- Stand straight with your feet shoulder width apart and your head straight and looking forward.
- Gently tilt your head to the right and start rolling back.
- Keep rolling your head to the left and then down.
- Bring your head up to the starting position and repeat in the opposite direction.

SHOULDER ROLLS

- Stand straight with your arms by your sides and with your feet shoulder width apart.
- Slowly rotate your shoulders forward, making big circles.
- Repeat the movement backward until the set is complete.

BIG ARM CIRCLES

- Stand straight with your feet shoulder width apart.
- Raise and extend your arms to the sides, without bending your elbows.
- Slowly rotate your arms forward, making big circles.

- Complete a set in one direction and then switch, rotating backward.

FLEXION/EXTENSION

- Stand straight with your feet shoulder width apart and with your arms by your sides, palms facing up.
- Roll your shoulders forward and bend your upper back forward like a caving-in position.
- Then return to standing position and roll your shoulders back, squeezing your shoulder blades. Repeat.

REACH AND PULL

- Stand tall with your back straight, abdominals engaged, shoulders relaxed, and feet about hip width apart. Reach your arms straight up toward the ceiling, keeping them in line with your shoulders.
- Breathe deeply as you drive your right knee up toward the ceiling while pulling your hands down and your elbows toward the sides of your waist.
- Return your right foot to the floor while reaching overhead again.
- Switch sides by driving your left knee toward the ceiling while pulling your arms down, then returning your left foot to the floor and reaching overhead. Repeat.

STANDING HAMSTRING STRETCH (LEFT AND RIGHT)

- Stand tall with your left foot a few inches in front of your right foot and your left toes lifted.
- Bend your right knee slightly and pull your abdominals gently inward.

- Lean forward from your hips, and rest both palms on top of your right thigh for balance and support.
- Keep your shoulders down and relaxed; don't round your lower back. You should feel a mild pull gradually spread through the back of your leg.
- Repeat the stretch with your right leg forward.

STANDING QUAD STRETCH

- Stand tall with your feet hip width apart, pull your abdominals in, and relax your shoulders.
- Bend your left leg, bringing your heel toward your butt, and grasp your left foot with your left hand. You should feel a mild pull gradually spread through the front of your left leg.
- Switch legs and repeat the stretch.

CIRCUIT 1: CARDIO

JUMPING JACKS

- Begin by standing with your legs straight and your arms to your sides.
- Jump up and spread your feet beyond hip width apart while bringing your arms above your head, nearly touching.
- Jump again, lowering your arms and bringing your legs together. Return to your starting position.

OPTION: SIDE-TO-SIDE JACKS

- Stand tall with your back straight, abdominals engaged, shoulders relaxed, arms at your sides, and feet together.
- Bend your left knee slightly while extending your right arm overhead and stepping your right leg out to the side.
- Return to the start position, standing tall.

- Switch sides by bending your right knee slightly, extending your left arm overhead and stepping your left leg out to the side; return to the start position and repeat side to side.

JUMPING ROPE (OPTION: BOUNCE IN PLACE OF JUMP)

- Pretend you're holding a jump rope, and skip the invisible rope.
- Try other types of footwork throughout the 30 seconds; for example, jump on two feet or alternate hops.

HEEL-TOE (OPTION: HEEL-TOE BOUNCE STEP)

- Stand with your feet about 1 foot apart and your knees slightly bent.
- Lift your left knee up and place your left foot with foot flexed (heel into the ground and toe up) in front of you, body slightly leaned over, and right arm bent forward in a running position and left arm and elbow back, adding a bounce to your movement.
- Bring your left foot back to the starting position.
- Lift your right knee up and place your right foot with foot flexed (heel into the ground and toe up) in front of you, body slightly leaned over, and left arm bent forward in a running position and right arm and elbow back, adding a bounce to your movement.
- Bring your right foot back to the starting position.
- Repeat the action with the opposite arms and legs, following with a bounce action.

SQUAT TO PRESS

- Put your hands in fist position facing each other and hold them in front of each shoulder with your elbows close to your body.

- Push back into your hips and keep your back straight to lower into a squat, holding your fists up in front of your shoulders.
- When your hips are below your knees in the squat, push both legs into the ground to stand up and at the same time press your fists into the air overhead by straightening your arms.
- Slowly return your fists to your shoulders. Repeat.

CIRCUIT 2: STRENGTH

ROMANIAN DEADLIFT TO ROW

- Stand straight up with your feet about shoulder width apart and hold your hands in fist position by your sides.
- With a slight bend in your knees, hinge over at the waist until your fists with your arms straight reach your knees, keeping your back flat and your core engaged and tight.
- Now with your hands in fist position, pull your elbows back and squeeze your shoulder blades.
- Lower your arms back down, then stand back up.
- Repeat.

TRICEPS KICKBACKS TO UPWARD PULSE

- Stand upright with hands in fist position, facing in. Keep your feet shoulder width apart and your knees slightly bent.
- Keeping your back straight, bend forward at the waist until your torso is nearly parallel with the floor.
- Keep your head up and your arms bent at your sides so that your arms are aligned closely to your body, forming a 90-degree angle. This is your starting position.
- Using only your triceps, exhale as you extend your arms fully backward, bringing them nearly parallel with the floor.

- Repeat this movement 5 to 10 times, then hold the last extension 3 seconds, then rotate your fists up toward the ceiling with your arms straight and quickly perform 5 to 10 short pulses up toward the ceiling.

HORIZONTAL WOOD CHOP
- Stand straight with your feet shoulder width apart and hold your hands together.
- With your arms straight, rotate your torso to the right and return to center. Repeat for 45 seconds.
- With your arms straight, rotate your torso to the left and return to center. Repeat for 45 seconds.

CIRCUIT 3: CARDIO

SQUAT TO KICK
- Stand facing forward with your chest up.
- Place your feet shoulder width apart or slightly wider. Extend your hands straight out in front of you to help keep your balance. Or hold your hands at chest level or place them behind your head.
- Bend at your knees and hips, sticking your butt out like you're sitting into an imaginary chair. Keep your chest lifted and your spine neutral, and do not let your lower back round.
- Squat down as low as you can, keeping your head and chest lifted. Keep your knees over your ankles and press your weight back into your heels.
- Keep your body tight, and push through your heels to bring yourself and kick forward with your right leg (alternate kicking legs for each repetition).

INCHWORM PUSH-UPS
(OPTION: INCHWORM TO KNEE PUSH-UPS)

- Sit on the floor resting on your hands and knees. Form a tabletop with your back. Your knees should be aligned directly under your hips and your hands aligned under your shoulders.
- Straighten your legs back behind you, one at a time, forming one line from your head to your toes, and resting your weight on your hands and feet with your arms fully extended.
- Perform a push-up.
- For optional version, with knees slightly bent at your comfort level, walk your hands and body out to a plank position, staying on your knees. Perform a push-up or hold the plank position for 3 seconds.
- Now walk your hands backward to your legs to the start position and stand up straight.

SUPERMANS

- Lie facedown on the ground with your arms out straight overhead on the ground and your legs out straight behind you.
- Everything should be relaxed and your neck should be in a neutral position.
- Then squeeze your glutes, back, and shoulders to raise your chest and legs up off the ground. Try to get your chest up as high as possible as well as your quads. Keep your neck in a neutral position.
- Hold yourself up off the ground for a set amount of time, then lower yourself back down.
- Keep your arms and legs straight as you lift but do not lock them out. Do not bend your knees to try to get your quads higher up off the ground.

- Make sure to really squeeze your glutes as you lift so your lower back doesn't do all the work. And also make sure not to shrug as you lift your upper body.

CRUNCHES
- Lie on your back with your knees bent and feet flat on the floor, hip width apart.
- Place your hands behind your head so your thumbs are behind your ears.
- Hold your elbows out to the sides but rounded slightly in.
- Tilt your chin slightly, leaving a few inches of space between your chin and your chest.
- Gently pull your abdominals inward.
- Curl up and forward so that your head, neck, and shoulder blades lift off the floor.
- Hold for a moment at the top of the movement and then lower yourself slowly back down.

CIRCUIT 4: STRENGTH

ROMANIAN DEADLIFT TO FLY
- Stand straight up with your feet about shoulder width apart and hold your hands in fist position by your sides.
- With a slight bend in your knees, hinge over at the waist until your fists with arms straight reach your knees, keeping your back flat and your core engaged and tight.
- Now with your hands in fist position, turn the insides of your fists inward, facing each other.
- Raise your arms out to your sides with your hands facing down, squeezing your shoulder blades together during the movement. Keep your back flat and your head neutral.
- Lower your arms to the starting position. Repeat.

ALT REVERSE LUNGE TO BICEP CURLS
- Holding your arms down by your sides, hands in fist position facing up, step one leg back into a reverse lunge.
- Lift your fists and fold up your arms in a full bicep curl motion, then step your leg back up to standing position.
- Alternate legs.

DIAGONAL WOOD CHOP (LEFT AND RIGHT)
- Stand straight with your feet shoulder width apart and hold your hands together.
- Rotate your torso to the right and raise your straight arms over your right shoulder.
- Then squat as you rotate your torso to the left and bring your straight arms diagonally across your body until they are close to your left hip.
- Then switch sides.

CIRCUIT 5: CARDIO

SQUATS (OUT/OUT/IN/IN PULSE)
- Stand facing forward with your chest up.
- Place your feet shoulder width apart or slightly wider. Hold your hands in fist position at chest level.
- Bend at your knees and hips, sticking your butt out like you're sitting into an imaginary chair. Keep your chest lifted and your spine neutral, and do not let your lower back round.
- Squat down as low as you can, keeping your head and chest lifted. Keep your knees over your ankles and press your weight back into your heels.
- Keep your body tight, and in squat position, take your right foot out farther than shoulder width, take your left foot out farther

than shoulder width, bring your right foot back to shoulder width, and bring your left foot back to shoulder width.
- Repeat.

MOUNTAIN CLIMBERS (OPTION: ADD A CHAIR)

- Start in a plank position with arms and legs fully extended. The optional starting position is to use a chair, placed in front of you, with you holding on to the sides of the seat for added stability.
- Keep your abdominals pulled in and your body straight. Squeeze your glutes and pull your shoulders away from your ears.
- Pull your right knee into your chest. As your knee draws to your chest, pull your abs in even tighter to be sure your body stays up and in the plank position.
- Quickly switch and pull the left knee in. Simultaneously, push your right leg back and pull your left knee in to your chest using the same form.
- Continue to switch knees. Pull the knees in right, left, right, left—always switching simultaneously so that you are using a "running" motion. As you begin to move more quickly, be in constant awareness of your body position and be sure to keep a straight line in your spine and keep your head up.

BICYCLE CRUNCHES

- Lie flat on the floor with your lower back pressed to the ground and your knees bent. Your feet should be on the floor and your hands behind your head.
- Engage your core muscles, drawing in your abdomen to stabilize your spine.
- With your hands gently holding your head, pull your shoulder blades back and slowly raise your knees to about a 90-degree angle, lifting your feet from the floor.

- Exhale and slowly go through a bicycle pedal motion, bringing one knee up toward your armpit while straightening the other leg, keeping both elevated higher than your hips.
- Rotate your torso so you can touch your elbow to the opposite knee as it comes up.
- Alternate to twist to the other side while drawing that knee toward your armpit and the other leg extended until your elbow touches the alternate knee.

PUSH-UPS (OPTION: PUSH-UPS ON KNEES)

- Position your body with your arms straight out, abdominals tight, holding your body in a plank position. For the optional variation, hold a plank position on your knees just like the inchworm push-up.
- Hands and arms should be positioned slightly below your shoulders, fingers pointed forward. Shoulders are pushed down away from your ears.
- Lower your body until your chest is an inch or two above the floor, elbows pulling back at roughly a 45-degree angle.
- Push your torso away from the ground until your arms lock, then repeat.

COOL-DOWN

BRING BOTH KNEES INTO CHEST AND ROCK SIDE TO SIDE

- Lie on your back with your knees bent and your feet flat on the floor.
- Gently bring one leg up and then the other.
- Interlace your fingers or clasp your wrists between your lower legs, just below your knees.

- Gently pull your bent knees toward your body, using your hands.
- While you're pulling, try to relax your legs, pelvis, and lower back as much as you can.
- Hold for two counts and rock gently side to side.
- Return your legs to the floor.

The following stretches are a sequence; each stretch rolls into the next.

FLAGPOLE STRETCH

- Lie on your back with your knees bent and your feet flat on the floor.
- Gently bring one leg up while the other leg is straight on the ground.
- Grab the back of your leg (hamstring) and pull it toward your chest as far as you can, keeping your leg straight.
- Gently bring your knee into your chest and then straighten your leg to the floor.

CROSS-OVER-SPINE STRETCH

- Lie down on your back, bend your knees, and plant your feet into the ground, with your arms down by your sides and palms facing the floor.
- Bring one knee up to your chest and grab the outside of your knee with the opposite hand.
- Pull your knee toward your opposite shoulder while keeping your head, back, and shoulders flat against the floor.
- Hold for 20 to 30 seconds, then lower your foot back to the ground.

FLOOR QUAD STRETCH

- Lie on your left side, ensuring that your body is in a straight line from head to toe.
- Bend your right knee and bring your foot back directly behind you so that you can hold it with your right hand. You should feel a stretch on the front of your right thigh. Hold this position for 20 to 30 seconds.

UPWARD DOG

- Lie with your face and chest on the floor, hands by your sternum, and push your body up.
- Open your chest toward the ceiling as you straighten your arms. Your gaze will go up slightly.
- Keep your legs engaged and drop your hips toward the floor. The only things touching the floor should be the palms of your hands and the tops of your feet. Push strongly into both.
- Keep your shoulders over your wrists and draw your shoulder blades down and toward your spine to create space between your shoulders and your ears.
- Release and lower your body back to the floor.

CHILD'S POSE

- With your hands and knees on the ground, sink back through your hips to rest them on your heels.
- Hinge at your hips as you fold forward, walking your hands out in front of you.
- Rest your belly on your thighs.
- Extend your arms in front of or alongside your body with your palms facing up.
- Focus on breathing deeply and relaxing any areas of tension or tightness.

SHOULDER STRETCH
- While in child's pose position, bring your right hand and arm under your left arm and hand and slightly rotate to the right.
- Repeat on the other side.

ROLL UP TO SHOULDER ROLLS
- Flex your feet or tuck your toes, and raise your hips into a Downward Dog position. Drop your head down toward the ground. Keep your arms straight and elbows relaxed. Try to lower your heels to the floor as your legs straighten, keeping your feet about one foot apart. Your body should be at a 90 degree angle, making a straight line from your heels to your hips, and another from your hips down your arms to your hands.
- Walk your hands back toward your feet and gradually roll your body to standing, one vertebra at a time. Your head should be the last thing to come up.
- Roll shoulder rolls at the top, forward and backward.

EXTENSION/FLEXION
- Stand straight with your feet shoulder width apart and your arms by your side, palms facing up.
- Roll your shoulders forward and bend your upper back forward like a caving-in position.
- Then return to standing position and roll your shoulders back, squeezing your shoulder blades. Repeat.

TRY MEDITATION

Everyone and anyone can learn to meditate, and I find that it's one of the best ways to de-stress at the end of the day. Whether you meditate for 10 minutes or an hour, it will help you relax and unwind. Meditation alters the physical structure of the brain, and those who practice regularly say that they are calmer and happier. Meditation allows you to focus on yourself, put your worries aside, and have the space to experience your feelings without reacting to them.

You can meditate absolutely anywhere, sitting up or lying down. Wear comfortable, nonbinding clothing, and find a quiet space that is removed from as many distractions as possible. Some people like to meditate in silence. Others like listening to chanting or soft music.

If you are new to meditation, don't be surprised if at first you feel more agitated than relaxed. You may be tapping into some feelings that you have been pushing aside. This agitated feeling is healthy, and as you get more comfortable with your feelings, you'll notice that you will be able to release them and relax.

Begin each meditation by dimming the lights, then closing your eyes and focusing your attention on your breathing—following the in-breath and the out-breath. Let your breathing be slow, full, and rhythmic. Notice when your attention is drawn to a thought, sound, sensation, or emotion. Simply allow it to be there without resisting it, then gently bring your attention back to the breath. If you find yourself judging any aspect of what you are experiencing—for instance, if you find yourself lost in thought and judge this as "wrong" or "bad"—just notice the judgment as another "thought" and bring your attention back to the breath. Then follow these simple instructions for a 4-minute meditation:

1. Sit or lie down in a comfortable position. Close your eyes so that you don't get distracted.

2. Breathe in for 4 counts through your nose with your mouth closed.

3. Hold your breath for 4 counts.

4. Exhale through your nose or mouth for 8 counts.

5. Repeat this practice for 4 minutes. As you master this breathing meditation, increase your practice by adding 4 minutes at a time.

To take your practice to the next level, use this breathing technique when you are listening to any one of the free meditation apps that are available on your phone or laptop, like Calm, Headspace, or Insight Timer.

Combine this breathing practice with a *mantra*, which is a word or group of words that you concentrate on during meditation. Some people believe that mantras have spiritual powers; I use them to push out the negative thoughts that sometimes swirl around my brain when I'm meditating. Some mantras have a literal meaning, while others do not.

When I'm stressed, I repeat the following mantra in my head as I breathe:

I am a light for life

Feel free to use it too, or create your own.

GET MORE/BETTER SLEEP

One of the main complaints caregivers share is that they are exhausted. Fatigue can be caused by the physical and mental challenges of caregiving, or from the fact that you probably aren't sleeping well. In the early stages you may be worrying about your LO and how caregiving is going to affect your life. In the middle stages your LO may start wandering at night, which will disrupt your sleep.

The bad habits many of us pick up along the way don't help either.

Eating too much food too close to bedtime keeps your body hot at night, making it hard to drop off to sleep. Limited physical activity during the day—like sitting around the house—doesn't give you the opportunity to use your muscles that release sleep hormones. And sleeping with the light on, or having even the smallest night-lights or electronic lights on in your room, may prevent you from getting the rest you need.

Another problem is fragmented sleep, which is what happens when you wake up in the middle of the night. This problem is easier to solve because the causes are almost always environmental—something you're doing or exposed to that you can control:

- Acid reflux caused by eating too late
- Room temperature being too hot or cold
- Dehydration
- Noise
- Sleeping with a pet
- Snoring/sleep apnea

In a perfect world, you should get at least seven consecutive hours of sleep, including the time it takes getting into bed, settling down, and falling asleep. Think of every hour short of that as forming a sleep debt that piles up each night. So, if you slept for 6½ hours last night, you're beginning your day with 30 minutes of sleep debt. When you go to sleep the following night, you first repay this debt from the previous night. That means even if you sleep 7 hours the second night, it only counts as sleeping for 6½ hours again. Eventually, you have to repay your sleep debt or you will get physically sick. A short nap during the day is one way to repay some of your sleep debt, so when your LO sleeps, take a rest, too.

If you have trouble falling asleep, try these tips:

1. You should be cool in your bedroom. If you're sweating under your covers, it's time to rethink your pajamas, thermostat setting, or bedding.

2. Limit exposure to bright lights for an hour before you go to sleep. That means turn off overhead lights and turn down the brightness on your screens—or even better, put them away altogether.

3. If you need an alarm to wake up in the morning, cover it with a dark towel so that the light it emits doesn't disturb you. Or use the alarm on your phone and turn your phone facedown.

4. If you snore, make sure your doctor knows. Sleep apnea affects more than sleep: it is connected to poor heart health, diabetes, and being overweight.

5. It's hard to sleep when you are listening for your LO's movements at night or sleeping in the same room. Take the stress off by using a baby monitor if you are not sharing a room with your LO. That way you can be assured that you will hear them if they need you. If you are sharing a room with your LO who snores, have them checked for sleep apnea. Breathing strips for them, and earplugs for you, will go a long way toward making nighttime quieter, and continuous positive airway pressure (CPAP) devices are covered by Medicare.

6. Don't look at your watch/clock/phone to check the time when you cannot get to sleep or if you wake up in the middle of the night. It really doesn't matter what time it is, and knowing may only make you more anxious.

7. Lastly, don't create more stress by worrying about the previous night and whether you'll have the same bad experience again. You are in control. If you follow these simple recommendations, your sleep will improve a little bit every night.

PICK UP A NEW HOBBY, OR CONTINUE ACTIVITIES YOU ENJOY

Even when I'm exhausted, I do not like to sit on the couch and do nothing. In my free time I'm multitasking, which doesn't sound relaxing, but it is for me. I love to learn new things. Reading, especially about history, is one of my favorite forms of stress relief. It keeps me calm because I'm completely engaged with whatever I'm learning about. When I go to the gym, I'm also reading. When I watch a movie, I'm also folding the laundry. I am never without anything to do. But that's me.

If what I do doesn't work for you, then you have to find the thing that does. Some people craft; others talk on the phone with their friends. It doesn't matter what you do with your time as long as you are doing you, and it continues to light you up. You may want to take your interest to the next level. If going to church boosts your mood, think about joining a Bible study group. Write inspirational quotes from the Bible in your binder. Listen to your favorite church music.

Art and music are also amazing de-stressors. If you can't make an in-person visit, you can virtually visit almost any museum or concert hall in the world right from your laptop or phone. Just Google a place you've always wanted to see and take in a virtual exhibition or performance.

Or try something completely new. And try it with your LO. They will help you keep the pace slow so you don't feel any pressure to master a new skill in a week. You may find that this activity—painting, puzzles, sculpture, or watching old movies—is the catalyst that takes your relationship in a new and positive direction.

Nurture All of Your Relationships

Staying in touch with friends and family—and making time to see them—may seem like a big ask, but take it from me, it's critical. First, you never know who will volunteer to be part of your team, and by maintaining lots of relationships, you will have a bigger field to choose from. Your friends and family can also provide emotional support and entertaining distractions from the day-to-day.

If you have intimate relationships, pay attention to those as well. I'll just say it: sex is a stress reducer. If you are caring for your spouse, remember that both of you have sexual needs and desires. These can be fulfilled in a variety of ways once you remember that you are creating a loving, respectful environment.

WORK ON YOUR RELATIONSHIP WITH YOUR LO

Family relationships are a mixed bag. Some are blessed and close; some were fraught with tension and animosity long before this disease ever showed up. Caring for a spouse will be different than caring for a parent, and different still if you are caring for someone outside your nuclear family. I've been a caregiver in the full range of relationships: for my aunt, my neighbors, my parents, and the strangers who hire me. Each time, I try to build or reset these relationships in a new and positive light, which makes the work much less stressful.

The tool that has helped me the most is my faith. When I tap into my spirituality and put my religion's tenets into everyday practice, it helps me cope with challenges as they come up. I have also been able to have better, less stressful relationships with my LOs by letting go of past hurts and embracing the idea that there is more to life than what I see before me.

This type of spiritual support is available to everyone—and it doesn't have to come through organized religion if that's not for you. Your cultural or religious beliefs may have influenced your decision to be a caregiver. In fact, many of the world's spiritual practices share a philosophy of responsibility and care for others, and the ways we interpret that philosophy influences how we approach familial obligations. Our beliefs also help us make sense of the disease and the caregiving experience. These factors will impact the way you view your LO, so that you can embrace a perspective that is more positive and forgiving. This new outlook will go a long way toward resolving relationship issues from the past. In turn, carrying an attitude of grace and forgiveness makes caregiving less burdensome.

My friend Amanda, who was a caretaker for her mother for two years, recently told me, "As much as the work was tiring, it was very rewarding. Even with her dementia, there was a joy in knowing Mom in a way that I hadn't known before. We also healed a lot of wounds. On a spiritual level it was unique and special. We were able to get beyond the typical mother-daughter relationship. I felt I got closer to her and it was helpful for me that we shared the same spiritual direction. I believe I've become a more patient, empathetic, open-minded person, and I certainly appreciate life on this earth more."

Religious organizations often have established support groups for caregivers, which usually combine spiritual teachings with socializing and therapeutic support. This blend may be exactly what you need to regroup and reframe.

MANAGE YOUR EMOTIONS AS THEY ARISE

One of my best practices for getting rid of stress was learning how to manage my emotions. I've never been one to scream at my patients because it is not only unprofessional, it doesn't serve me or the patient. You cannot change someone's behavior by berating them. And any release you get from yelling in the moment won't make you feel better a few minutes later. On the rare instances when I lose my temper, it only makes me feel ineffective. The stress comes when I stop listening and forget to be a problem solver, which happens when my emotions get the best of me.

I learned early in my career how to deal with my emotions as they come up, instead of repressing them. My go-to strategy is to identify my feelings and then talk them through as quickly as possible. I do that by looking at an *emotion wheel*. American psychologist Dr. Robert Plutchik proposed that there are eight primary and oppositional emotions that serve as the foundation for all others: joy and sadness, acceptance and disgust, fear and anger, and surprise and anticipation. His emotion wheel is shown opposite.[1]

The center circle contains our most intense emotions. The first ring outside the center contains our primary emotions, and their opposites are listed across from each other. As the rings pull away from the center, they contain the related, less intense emotions. The emotions that appear between the spears are a combination of the two primary emotions that surround them.

Use the wheel to examine how you are feeling in any given moment. The goal is to articulate your emotions in a healthy, productive, and constructive way, not a reactive one. Once you've identified your emotion, think about what events or interactions activated it. This

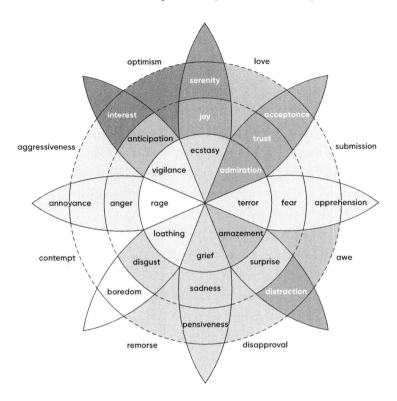

ability alone may empower you to express how you feel in ways that are in your control.

Psychoanalyst Mark Borg Jr., PhD, taught me that when someone doesn't understand their emotions, those emotions are acted out as a behavior, and often, a negative one. The problem is that emotions build on themselves and over time become more intense. Worse, acting-out behaviors don't release negative emotions; they only block your awareness of the underlying emotions. An emotion wheel helps us work our way backward from the acting-out behavior to its root cause.

There will be times when our behaviors toward our LO are not ideal. We may act in ways that are embarrassing and shameful, or even worse. When your emotions are roiling, step back and regroup with the emotion wheel: stop, identify your emotion, and find out what's driving it. Ask yourself, *Is it that I hate my LO? Is it that I'm sad? Is it that I'm old? Is it that I'm lonely? Is it that I'm losing my LO?*

As you look at the words in the center circle and move toward the outer circles, you may find that it's actually the softer, more vulnerable emotions that are driving your behavior. You don't necessarily act out loneliness in the same way you act out rage, but the rage may be the extension of the loneliness—unexpressed, unarticulated, unprocessed, and misunderstood.

Then approach your LO with the emotion wheel. It offers an easy way into a conversation to show them how you are feeling, discuss what happened, apologize, and move forward. Best of all, the wheel can help your LO express how they are feeling as well, even in the later stages of the disease when they are less verbal.

If you want to work with an emotion wheel on your own, ask yourself:

- What emotion am I really feeling?
- Why am I acting out?
- What do I need so that I don't act out again?
- Where am I going to find support for this emotional state that underlies my acting-out behavior?

LET GO OF STIGMA

In some cultures, and with some families, a dementia/AD diagnosis carries an enormous stigma for both the LO and the caregiver. Some believe that because AD has a genetic component, it brings bad luck to the family. Or there is a fear that if people in the community knew, they wouldn't want to associate with the family. Stigmatization is almost as dangerous as denial, and just as hard to get past. You can't be an excellent caregiver with this mindset. Worse, it's putting an extra burden on you. Keeping secrets hamstrings your ability to get the right programs, services, and healthcare for your LO, and for you. The fear of judgment almost always comes from not accepting one's condition. This is denial showing up once again. Knowledge is power. Educate yourself about this illness and its symptoms. The more you know, the less likely you will be to care what other people think. And then you will be free to get the best treatment and give the best care to your LO.

Connect with Your Community

If you were a member of a fraternity or a sorority in college, your local chapter, as well as the national organization, may run dementia/AD programs that provide resources, advocacy, and education. Check their websites and reconnect with old friends who may be in a similar situation. You can also start a group within your local chapter and share your experiences.

For communities of color, the 100 Black Men of America, the Center for Black Equity, Black Women for Wellness, The Links, and the National Council of Negro Women all have national and local chapters. The National Alliance for Hispanic Health and the Asian & Pacific Islander American Health Forum are national organizations that are community oriented. Or look directly at your local communities and see what support groups they provide.

JOIN A CAREGIVER SUPPORT GROUP

Your friends and family will hopefully support you throughout this caregiving journey. Yet they won't know exactly what you are going through, and it can be hard to share frustrations about other family members. A support group introduces you to other caregivers who are going through it, too. It is an opportunity to make new friends and get a deeper level of support, because they offer a safe space to share and discuss concerns, feelings, and experiences. You can also learn about other people's best practices and see how they may work for you and your LO. Lastly, a support group with people from your culture can reduce stigma on both the personal and community level.

Many religious groups and local nonprofits offer support groups. Check out the Alzheimer's Association and AARP websites for groups in your area. In the age of Zoom, you can join one almost anywhere without leaving your home.

WHAT'S NEXT

Feeling more confident? In the next chapter I show you how to make any home accessible for your LO. Creating the right environment makes caregiving a more pleasant experience, as you are removing potential risks and planning for disease progression.

CHAPTER 4

Organizing the Home

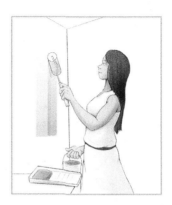

When I start working in a new home, the first thing I do with the family is reorganize the space. I always ask the family about the behaviors of the person I'm caring for as well as anyone else who lives with them. Then I make suggestions based on where they are at right now. For instance, the modifications I will suggest are likely different if their LO is already in Stage 5 versus Stage 3. I consider what kinds of pets they have and if they are still socializing where they need extra seating in the family room and dining room. One woman I cared for loved flowers, so I picked up fresh flowers for her every three or four days. The goal is to keep a house feeling like a home, while making it as safe as possible now and going forward so that you and your LO can remain there as the disease progresses.

As your LO moves through the stages of dementia/AD, the decline can be slow or very rapid. Your LO could be stuck in Stage 4 for a year or a week. This is why I suggest that you get the house in order as soon as possible. If you improve the environment before you need to, it will give everyone a chance to get used to the new space. And you are guaranteeing that you are providing a safe environment for your LO and yourself. As your responsibilities become more physical, you don't want to be tripping over—and potentially ruining—family heirlooms.

You also want to limit access to places where trouble can brew. I once worked with a retired couple where the wife had dementia. The husband didn't want to make changes to their home that he thought would upset his wife. He wanted to leave the stovetop alone so that the wife would think she still had the option to cook meals, even though I was doing all the cooking. However well-intentioned, this decision proved disastrous when the wife burned the teapot to a crisp because she forgot to turn off the gas burner.

I hold an Aging in Place certification from the National Association of Home Builders. What follows are the absolute best practices I have learned on the job and through this certification process. When you've made the recommended modifications, you and your LO will be able to stay in your home well into old age. And best of all, the cost of most of these suggestions is minimal.

A safer environment makes a huge impact on your stress level. The suggestions throughout this chapter will take away the worry of your LO getting hurt or of injuring yourself while providing care. With those two concerns taken care of, you can focus on sticking to your Family Care Plan and enjoying each day with your LO.

START WITH THE BIG PARE-DOWN

I've worked in thousands of homes, and the one thing they all have in common is that people, over time, collect a lot of stuff. I'm not going to point out any particular hoarders, but the truth is everyone's stuff needs to be organized, and some of it needs to be removed if you want to make a home safe. At the same time, you don't want to make the space so sterile that it doesn't feel like home. The secret is to find the balance between what you need and what you want. You are going to need to constantly reevaluate the way you and your LO use your home. What works this month may no longer work four or five months from now. However, once you have the paring-down mindset, it will be easier to let go of items that no longer serve you. This process will be much easier to accomplish before any health issues affect you or your LO. However, if that time has passed, it's never too late to start.

What you need refers to anything that makes you happy to look at that doesn't pose a risk of breaking or falling over it. Think of the most familiar, non-breakable items that make your house or your LO's house a home. Those will be the focal points in each room. Everything else can be packed away or given away, and the sooner the better: anything delicate or breakable that's out of your LO's home will be appreciated by someone else, who can keep it in good condition for future generations.

If your LO is in the earliest stages and isn't in denial, make the paring down an activity to do together. Set aside some time to look over every room, decide what is no longer needed, and which family members or friends would benefit from their things right now. Once your LO is in the moderate stages, their anxiety may prevent them from easily letting go of favorite objects. By the time my friend Rob's grandmother Muriel was diagnosed with dementia, his family had been living in complete denial for about five years. Yet once her symptoms were obvious, the grandchildren decided to take action. Muriel had been an interior decorator and had a beautiful apartment that was filled with knickknacks and delicate antique furniture. When the family was ready to make some modifications to the apartment, most of the furniture was ruined, and what was left wasn't safe. The uphol-stery on the sofas and chairs was falling apart or stained. The legs of the furniture became unstable because she wasn't able to gently get in and out of the chairs. None of it could be saved. Had they assessed her situation more realistically and sooner, the rest of the family could have moved these beautiful items into their own homes, where they would have been safely appreciated.

Since the furniture was already ruined, the grandchildren kept it in the apartment and focused on making it as safe as possible. They rearranged the furniture so that it was easier to maneuver around. However, there was one glass-topped coffee table that posed a safety threat. One day, when they were all at Muriel's home, they packed up the table right in front of her. Later Rob told me, "As we were put-ting the table away, she was crying and wouldn't talk to us. She was clearly very angry. We kept telling her that we didn't want anyone to get hurt, but she couldn't really understand why we were taking away her table. She was never someone who liked being told what to do, and she loved her things. It was an awful experience."

I told Rob that a better strategy would have been to remove the table when Muriel wasn't home. There was a chance that she wouldn't notice it missing. And if she did notice, he could have calmly ex-plained that the table was now being used by one of the grandchil-dren, or that it had been sent out for repair. The way he had chosen to do it was not only traumatizing, it was disrespectful, which was prob-ably why she was so incensed.

Keep this story in mind as you pare down. How you remove items is just as important as choosing which items have to go. Remember that you are making the right decision, even if it is painful. Stick to your plan.

Be sure to keep favorite pieces of artwork and photographs that trigger positive memories, but you may need to alter how they are displayed. The glass panels inside picture frames can easily be replaced with plexiglass, and the frames can be mounted on the walls. Limit the number of photographs so that your LO can focus on immediate family. It's likely that they will retain long-term memories far better than more recent ones, so photos of their parents and grandparents will also be appreciated. Display photos on the refrigerator with magnets; if they get pulled down, you can put them back up without risk to anyone.

SPEND MONEY ON HOME IMPROVEMENTS AND IMMEDIATELY REAP THE BENEFITS

Many families resist putting money into their homes to accommodate their LOs. Some have told me that they would rather use those dollars for hiring additional help. Others just want to keep their money in their own pockets, or they tell me that their LO would never have spent money on themselves. While those excuses may sound reasonable in the short term, I guarantee that they're never effective long-term strategies.

No one expects to develop dementia, so your LO may not have made their desires known about how to spend their money. While it may be hard to have conversations about money now, it's critical that you get clear that some money does need to be spent. The improvements that I will lay out in this chapter are there for only one reason: to make your LO safer and more comfortable.

Second, even though you think you're spending money on your LO, you will reap the benefits. These upgrades will make your life easier and less stressed, which in turn will make it easier for you to provide excellent care. The one thing all caregivers need to avoid is pain brought on from caregiving, and you shouldn't hesitate to spend on modifications that will make your job less physically taxing. The modifications that I've outlined are for the most part relatively inexpensive. Sell the stuff you're getting rid of on Craigslist or Facebook Marketplace, or donate it to a nonprofit for a tax deduction. See if you can borrow some of the recommended items from friends and family. Websites like Nextdoor and Freecycle are excellent ways to buy or sell used items right in your own neighborhood. Lastly, the "smart tech" items listed in the Home Technology Swaps section are not as expensive as you may think.

Not only that, any major improvements, like updating or enlarging a bathroom, will increase the value of the home. Today's real estate buyers are looking for homes that have the latest tech and are fully modernized. And if you do the work now, you can enjoy living in a better-functioning home for years to come, and profit from these updates whenever you are ready to sell. Some of the updates can also be tax deductible because they are considered "medical modifications." Keep your receipts and check with your LO's accountant before you file their taxes.

If you or your LO is over 65, you may qualify for senior grants from the federal and state governments to cover the costs of home repair and renovation. National charities often provide grants for seniors as well. For instance, the National Family Caregiver Support Program provides financial support for those caring for relatives age 60 or older, and you can use that money any way you like, including for repairs. Your church or house of worship can recommend volunteers in the congregation who are willing to help with major or minor home repairs, free of charge. Your community's Office of Aging may offer senior grants as well.

A WHOLE-HOME ASSESSMENT

Next, start looking at the home as a whole. Dementia/AD affects spatial perception, so the way your LO sees and moves through their home will change as the disease progresses. They may have a hard time differentiating between a floor and the steps to another level of the home. Or if a room's décor is all the same color family, they may not be able to pick up on the distinction between a wall and a horizontal surface, like a table.

These suggestions apply to any room of the home. For the most part, they are redecorating ideas that can be accomplished with just a few trips to the hardware store, and a handyman if necessary.

REVIEW FLOORING

All of the flooring in the home should have a nonslip, matte, or dull finish: glare from tile or polished floors can be disorienting and, when wet, slippery. Remove all loose area rugs. Matte tile decals are an easy way to cover existing flooring (like wood, vinyl, or tile) without the expense of pulling them up.

If you are replacing flooring, choose a material that has a texture, and a color that strongly contrasts with your walls. Avoid wavy lines and stripes. In general, all flooring for connecting areas should be in a similar coloring, even if the materials are different. When the floor colors are not similar, your LO may perceive the transition to be two different levels (causing them to try to step up or down) or mistake an actual transition for a shadow, which also leads to falls.

Options to consider include the following:

- Low-pile carpet (the ones "for commercial use" are easiest to clean)
- Wood floors
- Luxury vinyl flooring, which looks like wood and is easy to maintain
- Matte tile in a small format so there's lots of grout, which makes tile less slippery

LOOK AT YOUR LIGHTING

As all people age, the lenses in their eyes alter the way they perceive color and shadow. Shadows cause particular challenges. The long shadows thrown by natural light at sunrise or sunset may be distressing to someone with dementia/AD. One way to minimize shadows is to adjust your lighting to soft lighting from overhead fixtures. Small table lamps emit hard light, which casts more shadows and are more prone to breaking. Chandeliers are good choices because they bring overhead light closer to the objects in the room and further soften the light.

- All lighting controls on the walls should be labeled and in a contrasting color to the walls so that they are easily identifiable.
- People with dementia/AD often keep their gaze on the floor. Adhesive lighting strips positioned on floors can form a bedroom-to-bathroom walkway for nighttime use.

CHOOSE COLORS WISELY

One of the primary goals of excellent caregivers is to lower stress whenever possible. The less agitated your LO is, the better they will be able to comply with your directives. One way to keep stress to a minimum is to create a serene home environment. One trick I've learned is to decorate with a limited number of colors in each room and remove strong wallpaper or upholstery patterns. Think about the typical colors you see in newly remodeled homes. People often choose whites, beiges, or grays, and carry these colors on both the flooring (carpets, tile, wood, etc.) and the walls. However, for a person with dementia, this doesn't work. Even though it makes the room look larger, clean, and uncluttered, your LO will have difficulty determining where the flooring ends and the walls begin, leading to falls or accidents. Instead, use contrasting colors for floors, walls, and tables to help define vertical and horizontal surfaces. The walls can be white, but choose a darker floor covering and furniture that stands out from the walls and the floors. To draw attention to doorways, paint the door and the molding a different color than the walls. When setting the table, the color of the dishes should be in strong contrast with the tablecloth, place mats, and the table itself.

Colors are deeply personal, although there are some rules of thumb. Blues have a calming effect and are good choices for bedrooms. Greens are thought to reduce central nervous system activity and help people feel calm and rested. Reds and oranges can be agitating, so I don't recommend them as a first choice. However, if your LO is partial to a particular color, using it in your décor will make them happy.

Solid-color surfaces, fabrics, and walls (versus patterned) are easier for someone with dementia/AD to understand. For example, a speckled pattern on a dark background can be perceived as crumbs, which your LO may attempt to clean up.

DON'T FORGET THE WINDOWS

- Blackout shades effectively block out light for more restful sleep.

- Keep shades and drapes open during the day to allow natural light in, closing them at night to avoid reflections on the window and to indicate it is nighttime.

ROOM-BY-ROOM TIPS

If you have ever babyproofed a home, some of these suggestions will seem familiar or even commonsense, as every room in the home can pose a unique threat. Other changes address the specific needs of someone with dementia/AD.

CLOSETS

Some people with dementia like to empty closets and drawers. Your LO may start rummaging through cabinets, drawers, a refrigerator—any place where things are stored—in an attempt to find or even hide an item. This behavior is annoying to clean up after and can be hazardous. Once, when we were moving my neighbor to a smaller apartment, we found a set of dentures that she had accused me of taking behind the cleaning supplies.

Designate a lockable closet that only you can access to ensure that your LO won't hide anything inside. Store breakables there, as well as anything that could be dangerous, including cleaning supplies, medicines, sharp knives, and anything that is tricky to clean up or put back properly. It's an ideal location for valuables that could be misplaced or hidden, like legal papers, medical records, checkbooks, charge cards, jewelry, cell phones, and keys. I like to keep all my medical supplies and first-aid equipment in one or two large baskets inside the closet (see page 122 for my complete shopping list). This way, when there is an emergency, I can grab the whole basket and quickly attend to my client. Then designate another closet that is easily accessible for your LO. This is the place to store non-breakable items like sheets and towels, plastic containers, paper shopping bags, and shoes. Sorting through this closet could be an activity during the moderate stages. Your LO can store their meaningful yet safe possessions there, like photo albums.

KITCHEN

In the early stages of the disease, you should label the drawers, cabinets, and appliances in the kitchen. These labels will help your LO find items and put them away in the right spots, or give simple instructions on how to use an appliance, like the microwave. Be proactive with labeling because your LO will likely not skip this stage (in which they are still safe to use the kitchen but need some extra support), even if it's brief. The more attractive the labels, the more likely that they will not embarrass your LO or make them feel ashamed that they don't remember where things go.

By the time your LO is in the moderate stages, you will have to do more to make the kitchen safe and accessible:

- Your LO should not be using the oven/range/stovetop, and oven knob locks are essential to limit access. They may still be able to use the microwave to heat food, although in the later stages they may need help pushing the buttons.

- Consider your food storage containers and the packaging for anything you buy. Plastic containers and packaging are safer and lighter than glass.

- Take your LO's personality into consideration when you are deciding where to store sharp objects like knives. If your LO was always prone to violence, or if they're angry, argumentative, or combative, you don't want sharp objects around at all, and knives should be moved to your locked closet.

- Small appliances like coffeemakers and toaster ovens should have an automatic shut-off feature, or be moved to an inaccessible location or replaced with a newer model.

- Swap out fine china and ceramic dishes for plastic or melamine plates and cups. Choose nonslip items with bright colors; your LO may respond better to food on divided plates.

- Look for the Oxo brand "Good Grips" utensils, which are larger and weighted.

- Keep trash cans covered and, if possible, out of sight. Your LO may not remember what a trash container is for and either rummage through it or hide items inside. Always check your garbage before you empty it, just in case something has been hidden or thrown away by accident. I've had clients throw their wallets or important papers in the garbage, thinking it was a safe place to store personal items.

- Place a large kitchen clock with numbers on the wall so that your LO can see the time.

- In the later stages, purchase adult-sized bibs to protect your LO's clothing.

Emergency Info Poster

Create a poster/display with emergency information and often-used phone numbers printed in big letters. Make sure it includes your name and cell phone number, the names and phone numbers of your LO's children, their primary care physician, their health insurance company and policy number, the address of the home, and a list of any medications they may be taking. This information will come in handy if someone is covering for you and there is an emergency, or if your LO wants to call someone just to say hello. This poster should not include any vital personal information, like a Social Security number or a credit card, because as they progress in the disease they may answer the phone and be tricked into giving that information to a fraudster or someone preying on seniors.

LIVING ROOM/DINING ROOM/DEN

These rooms can continue to be used for watching television, working on activities, working out, eating meals, or socializing throughout the stages of the disease. This means that the more modifications you implement early on, the longer your LO will be able to be safe and comfortable in these spaces.

- People with dementia/AD sometimes open and slam cabinet doors, which can break the items inside. Lock the china cabinet so it's only a "display" to prevent this behavior.

- Clear end tables of knickknacks and replace with sturdy, decorative planters filled with live or faux plants and flowers.

- Arrange furniture so that there are clear paths that can accommodate walkers or wheelchairs.

- Replace cloth furniture. You don't have to invest in expensive or even new seating, but consider replacing your chairs and sofas with sturdy furniture that can be easily wiped down. Leather or vegan leather furniture is easy to clean, and easier to line with towels to prevent staining from incontinence or dropped food. Keep upholstery patterns simple, with minimal patterns, and choose colors that contrast with the floor and walls.

- If you are going to buy one big-ticket living room item, consider a power recliner that extends to full standing position. This type of chair will assist your LO in the later stages to move from sitting to standing. Recliners also help to eliminate painful swelling in the feet and infectious cellulitis, and they can lower the risk of heart disease. Bob's Discount Furniture and La-Z-Boy are two national chains that carry them. Medicare will pay for the motorized portion of a chair only if it transitions from completely sitting to completely standing. However, they will not pay for the whole chair; this is another reason why it's critical to understand the yearly Medicare rulebook.

- Label the television, radio/stereo, and smart speakers. Keep the television remote handy and always store it in the same space. Purchase extra remote controls: label them with numbers, program them, and store them in your locked closet for when one goes missing.

- Purchase washable activity boards and wall calendars and prominently display them in the living room or den where the activities will be taking place. Use them to write down a rough version of the week's Family Care Plan so that your LO sees what activities or chores need to be accomplished each day.

- Store similar items together and always in the same place. When I was taking care of my aunt, I made distinct sections in her living room, with books and magazines in one area and games in another.

- Consider a lightweight, adjustable TV tray for your LO to use for projects or meals. These can be carried from one room to another.

BEDROOM

The bedroom should have a calm atmosphere. When I redecorated my aunt's bedroom, I painted the walls a pale blue and the ceiling white just because I thought the combination was soothing. Later, I read an article in the *New York Times* that suggested that I was on to something: nursing homes in the Netherlands are being reimagined to provide people with late-stage dementia/AD a serene environment. They are finding that these lucky people need less medication to keep them calm day after day.[1] One strategy was to bring the natural world in: paint bedroom ceilings to look like a beautiful blue sky or add a mural on the walls with an outdoor scene. Even a large poster or painting of nature will improve one's mood and have lasting results.

Keep the furniture in the bedroom to a minimum. Your LO needs a bedside table or two, a dresser, and a television. You can use one of the bedside tables as your de facto workstation, so it needs to be large enough to hold your basket of medical supplies. And while they may not want to watch TV in their bedroom, you will probably be doing so during the latest stages when you need to keep an eye on them as they sleep.

The most noticeable change in the bedroom is usually the bed itself. In the early and moderate stages, your LO can continue sleeping in their bed as long as it's accessible on both sides (not placed against a wall) so that's it's easier for you to make the bed and change the sheets, and less aggravating for them if they can't find their way out of the bed. Position the bed so that your LO has a direct view of the bathroom during the night.

In the later stages, your LO should transition into a hospital bed, which is safer for them and easier for you. Position the hospital bed in the same place in the room so that you can easily get around three sides. A hospital bed is a twin-sized, motorized rental bed that elevates both the head and the feet. This configuration is critical not only for your LO's comfort: it will help you provide care without putting strain on your back. Your LO will require one when they can no longer stand up and get out of bed on their own, typically in Stages 6 and 7. Medicare will cover the cost.

When my own mother's health was declining, I ordered one because I knew that she would be more comfortable and it would be easier for me to take care of her. Because it was smaller than her old bed and we didn't have the right sheets, I bought new, pretty sheets to make it cozy, and she never felt like she was in an institutional hospital bed.

Making the Bed

Make up the hospital bed with beautiful sheets and blankets to make it homier. Contrast the bedding with the floor and wall colors so that the bed stands out in the room so that your LO can get to it safely.

Whether your LO is sleeping in a regular bed or a hospital bed, you need at least two sets of sheets, a comforter, an inflatable mattress pad, and a waterproof mattress protector. Consider purchasing a weighted blanket, which is not as heavy as the name suggests. A weighted blanket seems to have the same effect as swaddling a baby: it provides comfort and the feeling of a hug. I have seen it to be an effective tool for people with dementia/AD by helping them feel secure while sleeping, or even when they are sitting in a chair. However, they are not recommended for the latest stages, or if your LO cannot lift more than five pounds. At that point, you may also consider adding an air mattress on top of their existing mattress, which will prevent your LO from developing bedsores.

Limit the number of pillows on the bed; too many may be confusing for your LO. However, they may need additional pillows to place in between their legs or under their feet. If you want hospital-grade pillows for this use, do a Google search for *bed positioning aids*.

If your LO is sleeping in their own bed, line both sides with adult-sized bed rails that slip in between the mattress and the box spring or the frame. If your LO is a busy sleeper and their bed doesn't have a footboard, put a railing at the foot of the bed as well, install a footboard, or place additional pillows at the bottom of the bed. Drape the top sheet and blankets over the footboard and then tuck them under the mattress to keep them in place. This will form a tented area to improve airflow to the feet. Use additional pillows or a folded blanket to elevate the feet.

You will also need an additional flat sheet (or two, so that you have clean ones on hand) to use as a *draw sheet*. This sheet protects the flat sheet from soiling if your LO is incontinent, even if they are wearing disposable underwear to bed. It can also be used for repositioning your LO if you need to turn them so that they don't develop bedsores, or when they slide down too far into the bed.

First, lay the draw sheet over the entire bed, folding it in half from the bottom of the bed to the top. Fold it in half once more, placing it on the bed so that it sits where your LO's chest will be when they are lying down, extending to midthigh. The sheet should be completely flat: seams and wrinkles can irritate the skin. Then place a disposable pad and a reusable cloth pad on top. In the morning, if these sheets are soiled, throw away the wet disposable pad, wash the cotton pad and the draw sheet, and return them to the bed so that you'll be ready to go for the next night. In the next chapter, you will learn how to use the draw sheet as a transfer tool for getting your LO in and out of a bed or chair.

Other Small and Easy Upgrades to the Bedroom

- Humidifiers for dryness or air purifiers that remove allergens may help your LO get a better night's sleep.
- In the late stages, a bedside commode is useful to avoid complicated nighttime trips to the bathroom.
- Install motion sensors and a baby monitor, which will alert you to your LO's nighttime movements if you are sleeping in another room.
- Keep a mini fridge in the bedroom; you can even use it as a bedside table as it provides a large surface for your workstation. Keep a supply of cold drinks, like water bottles, handy to prevent dehydration.
- Attach a cup holder to the bedrail.
- Remove locks from bedroom doors.
- Keep facial tissues and a roll of paper towels by the bedside. Aside from their regular uses, you'll be needing them to clean up spills and when you are administering liquid medications, like eye drops.

BATHROOM

The bathroom is probably the most expensive remodel, but it's money well spent—and completely necessary. If you own your home, updated bathrooms that are compliant with the Americans with Disabilities Act (ADA) are a selling feature. In fact, new homes are built with bathrooms that follow these recommendations. If you are renting, tell your landlord that making these changes will ensure the safety of your LO. All of the ADA recommendations are appropriate for someone with dementia/AD, as well as few more:

- All-white bathrooms may be trendy, but they are confusing for those with dementia. If you are up for a complete remodel, choose darker colors on the bathroom walls so that the white fixtures (toilet, sink, shower/tub) stand out.

- If you install a new toilet, choose one that is taller than standard height, referred to as *comfort height*. If your LO is tall and requires a toilet that is even higher, build a permanent, decorative platform and install the toilet on top. There are also replacement toilet seats that sit right on top of your existing toilet to raise the seat as much as 3.5 inches.

- Install grab bars by the toilet and in the shower.

- If you are updating your shower/tub area, remove the existing tub and install a larger shower that is large enough to accommodate a seat. New showers can be installed as "curbless" so that the entrance is completely level with the bathroom floor. This is ideal for when your LO needs to be wheeled into the shower, in the later stages of the disease, and to prevent tripping. Inside, the shower floor is slightly pitched so that the water drains and doesn't enter the rest of the bathroom.

- If you cannot remove a bathtub, remove any glass sliding doors so that you can maneuver your LO with ease. A curved shower curtain rod with a waterproof shower curtain and liner is an ideal replacement.

- Install a handheld shower head for safety, cleanliness, and maintenance of the area.

- Bathroom doors are often smaller than regular doorways. Enlarge the door for wheelchair accessibility.

- Bathroom floors should be slip-resistant tile with a lot of grout lines for traction. Add non-skid decals to any slippery areas in the shower and the rest of the bathroom.

- Place a brightly colored, non-skid floor mat in front of the toilet, and add a bright toilet seat cover.

- Empty the medicine cabinet and put everything in the locked closet except for hairbrushes and toothbrushes.

HOME TECHNOLOGY SWAPS

Smart speakers, or virtual intelligent assistants like Amazon's Alexa and Google's Home, are ideal for an aging-in-place population because they allow control over the environment without getting out of your chair. They are also a source of information and entertainment.

As you renovate, make your home as tech friendly as possible, which means investing in the latest "smart" technology. Smart home systems use voice control and can be connected to other electronics in the home, including the following:

- Bathroom scale
- Deadbolt/lock
- Doorbell
- Home security system
- Indoor/outdoor lighting
- Robotic vacuum and mop
- Small kitchen appliances
- Smart plugs (which convert any small kitchen appliance into a smart appliance)
- Soundbars
- Surveillance camera
- Television
- Thermostat

Ironically, making your home smarter also means that your LO will need some old-fashioned equipment. As much as we love our smartphones, they are useless and frustrating for people with dementia/AD. That means that every app on their phone needs to be replaced with a physical item in the appropriate room. Don't fret about the expense: you don't need to invest in new versions. You may be able get some of these items from a friend, or purchase them used through eBay or other resellers. Once your LO enters the next phase of decline, some of them will no longer be of use.

Your LO may need the following:

- A corded or cordless telephone with oversized buttons. I recommend a corded phone that won't get misplaced.
- A large-print phone book
- A large calendar
- A radio/receiver/CD player/DVD player
- A large calculator
- Books and magazines

MUST-HAVES TO MAKE YOUR LIFE EASIER

Once you have the home reorganized, and in some cases renovated, the next step is to gather the tools you will need to be an effective caregiver. In later chapters, I will share how to use each of these items.

If you haven't familiarized yourself with the latest Medicare handbook, now is the time. You can find it online (www.medicare.gov), and it's also mailed to recipients every year. Understanding this document will help you plan what your LO may require for each stage.

If your LO already has Medicare, review their health and drug coverage and change their enrollment options if it no longer meets the needs of someone newly diagnosed, or if your LO could lower their out-of-pocket costs. Your LO doesn't need to sign up for Medicare each year, but you should still review their options annually. For example, according to the Alzheimer's Association, people with younger-onset Alzheimer's (also called early-onset) are diagnosed before the age of 65, and are eligible for Medicare once they have been receiving Social Security disability benefits for at least 24 months.

Medicare covers many costs associated with doctors and other healthcare providers, hospital stays, hospice care, home healthcare, skilled nursing facilities, preventive services, and prescription drugs. It also covers durable medical equipment (DME). Your LO will absolutely require some DME as the disease progresses. There are items for which Medicare will cover the majority of the cost when a Medicare-enrolled doctor or healthcare provider orders them for use in the home. These are ordered from a supplier that participates in Medicare and will process the paperwork—local medical supply stores, local hospitals, or online vendors.

The following list includes the items that Medicare covers, and when it is likely that your LO will need them. Note: not everything is listed in the Medicare handbook. In fact, there are a lot of items that are not in the handbook that Medicare may cover, but they won't let you know unless you ask. Many can be either rented or purchased from a participating supplier.

- Air mattress—moderate stage if they are already spending a large part of the day in bed. A medical air mattress is not the same as a blow-up mattress people use as a spare bed. It is a pressure-reducing support surface so that bedsores and wounds do not develop when your LO is lying in one position for too long.

- Bedside/portable commode chair—moderate stage

- Hospital bed—moderate/late stage

- Motorized lift—late stage, or earlier if your LO is already in a wheelchair

- Raised toilet seat—moderate stage

- Sit-and-lift mechanism for a power recliner—late stage unless your LO is arthritic or has other back issues, for which they may qualify earlier. Medicare will pay for the mechanism, not the entire cost of the chair. In this instance, you buy the chair from a retailer, and you will have to process the paperwork.

Other items that you will need that are not covered by Medicare can be purchased from a medical supply store or online. I'm amazed at how many big businesses, like Walmart and Amazon, have started carrying what used to be considered specialty items.

- Absorbent pads—moderate stage for use on a bed. In the later stages, you may have to cover living room/dining room furniture as well. These pads come in two varieties: reusable cloth pads that can be washed, or disposables. Another option is disposable dog training pads: they are exactly the same pads, just cheaper.

- Bath and shower safety mats—moderate stage

- Shower chair/bench/bath seat—moderate stage

- Slip-resistant, antibacterial, disposable toilet floor mats in a contrasting color—moderate stage

WHAT'S NEXT

At this point you have all the tools you need to prepare for caregiving. The second part of the book contains the critical lessons of the day-to-day experience. That doesn't mean that you should take the focus off yourself. Hopefully, you've learned that you can't afford to get lost in the shuffle. By mastering the best tips and tricks that professionals like me use, you can make caregiving far easier and more enjoyable.

PART II

Caregiving with Care

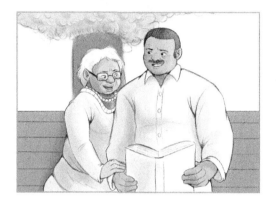

CHAPTER 5

Caregiving and the Activities of Daily Living

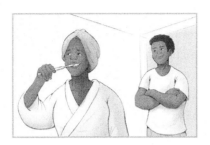

As a professional caregiver I'm always prepared, I anticipate my client's needs, and I provide the right services at the right time. The Family Care Plan you started in Chapter 2 allows you to develop these same anticipatory skills by scheduling team members so that your LO's needs are met before small problems become disasters. For instance, if you see that your LO is struggling to dress themselves, you'll schedule the occupational therapist to come up with solutions. When you respond in a timely manner, you will experience more joy and less burnout because there will be fewer daily surprises that cause you to feel physically and emotionally drained.

Every day will begin with the exact same structure: you will wake up an hour before your LO and get yourself ready. Then wake up your LO and begin the ADLs. I assure you that they are easy to master, and over time they will become second nature, as long as you develop the best-practice habits early on. Once they are done, you will be ready for the fun activities or appointments that are built into your Family Care Plan.

THE DAILY OBSERVATION

Your job as a caregiver is not only to keep your LO safe but also to help them achieve the highest level of functioning with peace and dignity. Nurses like me are trained to step outside a care situation and look at the patient objectively. I know that keeping an objective perspective is a big ask for family members or friends, but it is a skill that can be taught. What's more, having this ability will make you a better caregiver; you will be able to accurately convey changes in your LO's health to your team and tweak your Family Care Plan so that your LO feels successful and thriving, rather than frustrated or bored.

Being objective means that you are working from data instead of a gut instinct. In this case, your data is your LO. Every day you will be collecting information as part of your Daily Observation. With that data in hand, you can confidently adjust your strategies or leave notes for anyone who will be covering. Every day you will write some bullet points on how the day went. As you record your notes and review the ones you've made on previous days, you will be able to spot a recent decline, a change in behavior, or a physical situation that needs medical attention.

As your LO progresses into later stages, they lose their ability to tell you how they are feeling. If they usually like a hamburger for lunch, there will come a day when they refuse to eat it. They may not be able to tell you why it no longer works for them. It may be that they just don't feel like one today, and if that's the case then it's not a big deal. If you notice a pattern, it may mean something else is going on. It's possible that they no longer feel well after eating a burger, or that swallowing has become painful. Not only that, people with dementia/ AD are often living in the past. They may stop responding to their name and respond only to a childhood nickname. By collecting data, you will be able to pick up on issues like this even when your LO's ability to communicate is impaired.

The Daily Observation also helps to lower your stress level when you are at a doctor appointment. You don't ever want a doctor to ask you a question about your LO, and all you can say is, *"I don't know. I don't remember."* That's stressful. Instead, you want to be able to say, *"Since we saw you last, I've noticed these changes. We're definitely moving from stage 1 to stage 2,"* or, *"Happily, I haven't noticed any decline."*

FILLING OUT A DAILY OBSERVATION

It can be tricky to know what to look for in terms of signs and symptoms of deteriorating health. The best way to do this is to address symptoms on a daily basis. Professional nurses are constantly assessing people, and one of their protocols is to always record what they see in a chart. This is a simple tool that enables you to look for and track even the subtlest changes in health.

Use the following chart for your Daily Observation, or personalize one to meet your LO's needs. Fill it in at the end of each day, taking into account your LO's current abilities and medical and personal history. Every so often, go back to Chapter 1 and review the hallmarks of the dementia/AD stages. You are looking for mental declines as part of the assessment. Physical changes may not be related to dementia at all, but to other underlying conditions. Or their dementia may complicate the other health issues, because they're forgetting to drink or eat.

Assess your LO's status and health in the following context:

- *Describe Behavior/Task:* The desired behavior for the LO
- *Measure:* How much, how long, how far, and so on
- *Conditions:* The conditions under which the behavior should occur
- *Time Frame:* Whether the behavior was performed at the right time and for the right duration
- *Details:* Record your observation, with as many details as possible. This will help you see trends in what has worked, and what hasn't.

For example, one entry following breakfast could be "Mom sat down for breakfast (conditions). She ate (behavior) 2 eggs, a piece of toast, and a cup of black coffee (details) for 10 minutes (time frame). We were able to get to the table dressed and ready for the day in a timely manner (measure)."

Keep your expectations aligned with the reality of the disease. Just because your LO could button their shirt yesterday does not mean that they will be able to do it today. If you notice a switch, mark it down. Sometimes skills that they've dropped do come back. Other times, they are gone for good. It's easier to focus on short-term outcomes instead of long-term goals.

At the end of the day, record the best thing that happened. These will be your priceless moments, what I call Today's Joy. Later, reviewing them will remind you of your time as a caregiver.

Daily Observation: How Did the Day Go? Date:	
Activity	**Notes**
Bathing/dressing	
Breakfast	
Lunch	
Dinner	
Hydration: how many glasses of water?	
Exercise	
Activities	
Medical appointments	
Medication changes	
Behaviors: specific problems and overall mood	
Sleep	
Changes to the body (daily view): • Appetite • Sensory issues: dental, vision, hearing • Skin: tone, texture, wounds, sores, burns • Toileting issues	
Monitoring health weekly: • Blood pressure (if they are taking medications to control heart disease and vascular health) • Weight loss/gain	
Today's Joy	

Your Daily Observations Help You Flourish

You are flourishing in your role as a caregiver when you feel good about yourself, the work you are doing for your LO, and your relationship with them. Charting your Daily Observations will help you get there. Your notes provide a look back at the end of each day to see what small tweaks you can implement to make tomorrow more pleasurable. The truth is, when you feel like life is good, you are automatically providing better care.

As you review your Daily Observations, ask yourself:

- How do I feel about the job I'm doing?
- What accomplishment can I celebrate today? Is it the same as Today's Joy?
- What am I thankful for?
- What can I try differently tomorrow?

MEDICAL SUPPLIES TO HAVE ON HAND

These items should be kept in one or two large baskets in the locked closet, so that everything you may need is handy, and kept safe from your LO.

- Adhesive bandages for wound care
- Alcohol wipes to sterilize tools
- Aloe vera cream, petroleum jelly, or antibiotic ointment for treating wounds and burns
- AZO for treating urinary tract infections
- Basin for sponge baths

- Digital blood pressure monitor (upper arm or wrist cuff)
- Digital scale that calculates body mass index (BMI) and water hydration
- Disposable oral care swabs to keep your LO's mouth and lips moist during the late stages, when they are bedridden
- Disposable rubber gloves
- Extra batteries for digital tools
- Gauze pads for wound care and general cleaning
- Gel ice packs (keep in freezer)
- Hand sanitizer
- Hydrogen peroxide for cleaning wounds
- Nail clippers and nail file
- Otoscope: this device allows you to look into your LO's ears to see if there is wax buildup. You can use this once or twice a month.
- Pain reliever: Tylenol, Advil, or Aleve
- Pulse oximeter: measures oxygen saturation if you suspect COVID infection.
- Sheepskin products to relieve bedsores
- Skin cream or ointment containing zinc oxide to proactively create a protective barrier where pressure sores are likely to develop
- Soft mouth rest to aid in brushing your LO's teeth
- Tongue depressor: to check for redness or infection in their throat, like thrush (white lesions that can appear on the tongue, inner cheeks, tonsils, and roof of the mouth)
- Touchless thermometer
- Traditional stethoscope: can determine heart rate or if there is fluid in the lungs. It can also be used as a backup for your digital monitoring devices if the batteries run out.
- Washcloths (two at a minimum) for sponge baths

> **How to Take Your LO's Blood Pressure**
>
> Take your LO's blood pressure reading as soon as they wake up in the morning. If their blood pressure tends to fluctuate, they should be checked twice a day: in the morning and again after dinner. To get an accurate reading, make sure your LO is relaxed and that their arm is in a stable position. Follow the instructions that come with the monitor.

ADDRESS CONCERNS BASED ON YOUR DAILY OBSERVATION

Using your notes, you can draw inferences and reach a conclusion about any problems and devise a plan to address them. Then you can implement the plan and evaluate its effectiveness. If you notice that your LO is suddenly starting to nap during the day, try to determine why they are tired. Was there a change in medication? Are they not sleeping well at night? Are they becoming easily fatigued after physical activity? Are they dehydrated? Replace one potential trigger at a time until you determine the root cause. Chapter 8 has specific suggestions for dealing with the most likely health issues.

If the problem is consistent or not responding to your attempts to address it, contact your LO's primary care doctor. They will let you know if your LO needs to come in for an evaluation, or if they require additional assistance from another team member. Your Daily Observation will help you communicate vital information to both the doctor and your healthcare team. For instance, your LO may need the following special service providers. Your primary care doctor or you, depending on your insurance, can arrange for these specialists to provide assistance:

Physical therapy: If you notice changes to the way your LO is walking, such as less steadily, shuffling, limping, or pulling to one side, or if they are having radiating pain when they are moving their shoulders or lifting up their legs, difficulty standing or sitting, or any other kind of physical disruption in their daily movement.

Occupational therapy: If you notice changes in the way your LO is feeding themselves or getting dressed in the early to moderate stages. An OT provides tools so that your LO can continue doing the ADLs on their own.

Speech/language therapy: If you notice changes to speech or swallowing.

Nutritionist: If you notice consistent changes to your LO's bowel movements or swallowing, a nutritionist can make suggestions about changing up their diet.

TWEAKING THE FAMILY CARE PLAN

The Daily Observation allows you to collect data for implementing and adjusting the Family Care Plan. Having dementia/AD is the opposite of learning: you aren't going to see big leaps in improvement in a disease that only has one trajectory, which is downward. However, a flexible Family Care Plan can provide an overall sense of calmness and acceptance when a decline occurs, which makes your LO easier to be around.

Each time your LO shifts in abilities, discuss it with them in a context they can understand. Doing so will also help you understand their experience. You can explain why the daily structure is changing to include an afternoon nap, or a shorter activity. Get their feedback for as long as they can share it with you: your following their lead will help them feel like they have a little more control, which results in less anger and anxiety.

THE CARING HEART

Your Family Care Plan and Daily Observation are tools that influence each other.

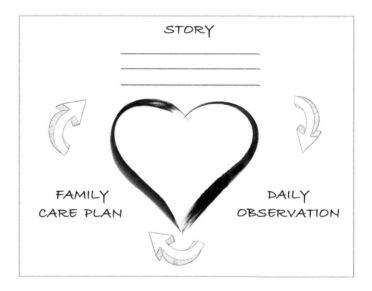

In the center of the heart, put your LO's name. At the top of the heart, under the word *Story*, list your LO's most definable characteristics. These are the aspects of their personal history that you need to take into consideration when you are planning their day-to-day routine. These aspects include religion, culture, education, standard of living, and overall lifestyle. Think about their personality, sense of humor, hobbies, favorite foods, and so on, and how you can incorporate them into the Family Care Plan; this influences everything from what you prepare for lunch to which activities to try. There may also be detrimental factors in their story: factors that can lead to setbacks or depression. These include previous health experiences, other underlying health issues, age, genetics, poor coping skills, and past traumas.

Your LO's story also influences your Daily Observation: how you will tailor their care as well as your expectations of their abilities and needs. The Daily Observation influences the Family Care Plan as your LO loses specific abilities over time; you will have to adjust the care plan accordingly. Ultimately, the Family Care Plan influences their story, as these aspects of themselves can either improve or decline based on the quality of your care.

MOVE THROUGH THE DAY WITH CLEAR COMMUNICATION

Taking the right approach when talking with your LO is probably the most important lesson in this entire book. Every caregiver will be able to quickly master how to get their LO cleaned, dressed, and fed, but it takes time and patience to put aside old familial roles and lovingly give directives instead of asking for permission or responding in anger every time something needs to get accomplished.

If it hasn't happened already, there will come a day when it is clear that your LO can't understand a direct question or follow a conversation. This could happen toward the end of the early stages. Even when your LO is engaged in a conversation, it doesn't mean that they understand what is being said. I once attended a family barbecue with my client Bella. We sat in one corner of her niece's backyard, and over the course of the party, her friends and relatives would come over and talk with her for a few minutes. Yet as soon as they walked away, Bella would stare off into the distance. When I asked her what was going on, she repeated the first line of the previous conversation. Bella couldn't follow in real time what her relatives were talking about. Later, when we returned home, Bella asked me to tell her about the party. She was hoping that I could explain what her friends and relatives were talking about.

When I pick up on this particular cue, my strategy immediately changes. I no longer ask a client for permission or give them a list of options before doing something. Instead, I switch to telling them what needs to be done in a gentle, loving way. While it may sound harsh, in reality you are making your LO's life easier by removing the threat of confusion or a confrontation. Your LO may realize that they are losing their independence when you switch to giving directives, but if you use the right tone, they will accept a role reversal more easily, and feel supported and less anxious. More importantly, giving directives allows you to remain in control. The truth is, people with dementia/AD can be addressed the same way we address children: lovingly, clearly, and with authority.

The second strategy that exceptional caregivers use to communicate is that they do not perform a task without letting their LO know what will happen next (as in, *"I'm going to give you your breakfast in a few minutes."*). When you say what you're about to do, you can see their anxiety noticeably diminish.

To make any directive more palatable, I accompany it with a physical touch. I have found that my clients respond more positively when directions are given with a loving touch or a soothing hug. This is true regardless of what stage they are in. Everyone likes to be reminded that they are loved. For example, if you want to get your LO out of bed, gently place your hand on their arm or the top of their head, and clearly say, *"It's time to get up."* As they sit up, rub their arm or give them a hug to motivate them; you may have to repeat your directive as you continue to comfort them: *"You have to get up. You have to get up."*

In the early to moderate stages, your LO may be defiant in response to your directives. Some of this behavior has to do with the dementia, which causes their personality to intensify. In my experience, if your LO was ornery before, they will be more difficult with dementia; if they were kind before, they will be kinder with dementia. Or they may not want to participate in the activity or task you are suggesting. They may even be more confrontational if they have nothing to look forward to, or if they are not socializing enough with peers.

Keep a copy of your Family Care Plan in the bedroom or the room where you will be spending most of your day, and point directly to it to remind them why they need to transition from one activity, like getting out of bed, to another, like getting dressed. When your LO sees that you have structured their day with interesting opportunities, they will be more likely to follow your instructions. Then incorporate your day's schedule into your directives. You are not only keeping them on track in the moment but preparing them for what's to come. For example, you can say,

"Let's look at the Family Care Plan and the weather to see what we should wear today."

Frame directives as part of a larger narrative. Connect an experience from their past and bring it into the present with a prompt for the task you want them to accomplish. For example,

"Last week you had a turkey sandwich at Joe's picnic and you loved it. I made the same delicious sandwich for lunch. Let's go into the kitchen and eat."

As your LO moves into the later stages of the disease, your directives will get shorter. Keep communicating throughout the day even if your LO is not responding verbally; just because they have dementia doesn't mean that they cannot hear you or appreciate the conversation. Even in the later stages, when they are less able to communicate, being clear in your instructions keeps them aware that something is going to happen.

PATRICIA'S TOP FIVE TIPS FOR COMMUNICATING

1. Set a positive mood before any interaction. Smile and make eye contact, and talk about something related to the interaction that they have enjoyed in the past.

2. Get your LO's attention. It's not particularly kind to yell a directive across a room. Walk up to your LO, look right at them, put your hand on them, and say their name and the directive clearly, using short sentences. For instance, *"Tom, it's time to get in the shower."*

3. If your LO is nonverbal, they may be sending you a message through body language. Look for their response with your ears, eyes, and heart. Your LO may not be able to find the words to answer you as quickly as you would like. Watch their eyes to see if they react to what you're telling them. Their eyes will convey their emotions and ability to understand.

4. Identify trigger words. Communicating is easier when you fully know your LO, including their history. Sometimes a hostile response has little to do with you; they may be locked on a memory that's related to the upcoming task, or a separate trauma from early in their life. When you have a better understanding of who they are as a person, you will be able to anticipate their reaction or figure out a better way to motivate them so you don't have to manage an aggressive response. For instance, when I learned that my aunt and her siblings had been placed in foster care when their mother died, I was able to avoid trigger words that would agitate her.

5. When the going gets tough, offer an incentive. My go-to is food. Suggest an outing to get a treat, or give them one in the home. You can also bribe your LO with an activity, such as art or music, as in, *"Tom, if you get in the shower now, I'll turn on some music while you get ready."* Or distract and redirect. *"Tom, tell me about that painting in the bathroom."*

THE TRUTH ABOUT TELLING THE TRUTH

When it comes to Alzheimer's or dementia, honesty is not always the best policy. I see so many family members argue with their LOs over the details of the past, or get themselves locked in a conflict about what's "real." It's all for nothing. You will never be able to force them to abandon their version of an incident or join the real world, and trying to do so only causes confusion, pain, anxiety, fear, and anger.

Instead, try what I call *beneficial fibbing* to spare everyone from unnecessary upset and distress. It's as simple as it sounds: a little lie to move a process or a conversation along, and include a distraction.

Here's an example:

Your LO says, *"I'm not hungry; I already ate lunch."* The truth is they haven't eaten in hours, and you have just prepared lunch. Gently say,

"Come to the kitchen for your afternoon snack. Let's eat it now because we have a busy day ahead of us."

You May Have to Introduce Yourself . . . Daily

Toward the end of the moderate stages and into the late stages, your LO may wake up confused and be startled seeing you, even when you've been living together for some time. Don't hesitate to start any conversation by introducing yourself with a smile and a touch. Try something like, *"Mom, good morning; it's your daughter, Tina."* Your LO will instantly feel relaxed as they may have recognized your face but forgotten your name.

NOTE HOW OTHERS TALK TO YOUR LO

While you're in tune with your LO's cognitive status, other people may miss the cues entirely, resulting in hurt feelings and worse, poor care. For instance, if your LO's doctor does not typically treat people with dementia/AD, they may not understand exactly what's going on with them. This is one reason why it's critical to have a doctor on your team who fully understands this disease, and why you as the caregiver need to attend all doctor appointments.

When I first started caregiving for my aunt, I accompanied her to all her doctor visits. At the time, I wasn't happy with the amount of medication she was taking. One day, as we were walking into the office,

I noticed that she became agitated, and by the time the nurse came in to take her blood pressure, it was significantly elevated. When the doctor came in, he started talking in a clinical way about her high blood pressure and prescribing even more medication. By this point my aunt completely froze, which was odd, because my aunt always had a lot to say. At the end of the appointment, I took the doctor aside and said, *"The way you talk to her is stressing her out. Her blood pressure is much lower at home. She just gets worked up when she sees you."*

The following week I found a new doctor and moved my aunt into a geriatric medical practice. I could see immediately that the new doctor understood how to talk to patients with dementia. She was soft-spoken, and when she talked to my aunt, she rolled her chair over and held her hand and made eye contact. She asked her short, direct questions. When the doctor saw that my aunt couldn't answer them, she reframed the questions to make them even simpler. At those visits, my aunt's blood pressure never went up and the doctor didn't recommend additional blood pressure medication.

HOW TO TREAT YOUR PARENT
WHEN THEY ARE ACTING LIKE A CHILD

Your role as a caregiver is going to change as your LO declines, until you eventually take on a parental role for your father or mother, spouse, or sibling. This adjustment is easier when you understand the disease and get yourself out of denial, and it happens in stages as the disease progresses. The truth is, once your LO is in the moderate stages, it's not in their best interest for you to try to maintain old roles.

However, you can still think of them as a loved one who needs your assistance. And because they are your LO, you don't want to make them feel ashamed or embarrassed when they make a mistake.

At first, you can take on the role as the behind-the-scenes fixer. For instance, if you see your LO buying more fresh food than they can possibly eat in a week, give some of it away or take it to another friend or relative. You don't have to chastise them publicly or privately, because they will probably not be able to learn from the experience. In short: you see a problematic behavior, and you accommodate for the behavior.

As the disease progresses and their abilities decline, you're put in the position where they relinquish control, and you pick it up. In other words, you are fully switching roles to become the parent, now treating them not like you would treat any child, but in the loving way you would treat your own child. You never want to argue with them or intimidate them. You're just going to keep the day moving forward through the Family Care Plan.

Once you take on the role of the parent, don't be surprised if the rest of the family starts to treat you like the matriarch/patriarch your LO used to play. And don't be concerned that your LO will feel bad relinquishing this role. In truth, you are taking some of the stress off their shoulders, which they will appreciate, whether they can express it or not.

MASTERING THE ACTIVITIES OF DAILY LIVING

If you are fortunate enough to be caregiving for your LO in the earliest stages, ask about their preferences when it comes to grooming and dressing. So many of my clients have family members who don't talk to their LO about the intricacies of day-to-day life and end up making decisions for them that don't make them happy. Or they wait too long to ask these questions and miss the opportunity for the LO to express their wants and desires.

Once your LO is in the moderate stages of dementia/AD, they will likely need your help with self-care. The clues for when this level of care is needed are subtle: Their home may not be as tidy as before. You may notice that their clothes are not pristine or they're wearing the same outfit every time you see them. All of these point to the fact that your LO isn't remembering to take care of themselves or their surroundings. These signs occur much earlier than problems with toileting or an inability to follow instructions, like taking medicine. However, they still need to be addressed quickly. By making small changes, you may be able to save some semblance of independence for your LO for a little while longer.

Helping someone with the activities of daily living is not the same as doing them for yourself. In fact, there is an absolutely right way to do them when you are caregiving. First, incorporate all the communication tools we've discussed as you move through the activities of the day. Remember to always break down actions into a series of steps, and remind your LO what's going to happen before each step takes place.

ADL caregiving will be challenging at first, because your LO may feel embarrassed, uncomfortable, or vulnerable, and in the later stages they may be afraid of you, who they perceive as a stranger. Approaching them with kindness, patience, and respect will make every aspect of care less stressful.

Getting the Team on the Same Page

This section is filled with tips and tricks that only the best-trained caregivers know. Once you have mastered them, share these life hacks with everyone in your family, especially those who are on your weekly team. When you have done so, everyone will approach caring for your LO in the same way.

Sharing this information within the family can be its own challenge. When I was taking care of my aunt, my main obstacle was one of her sons. He just could not get on the same page regarding her care and never listened to my advice. Ultimately, his refusal wasted time: I had to literally clean up his messes on the days when he took over the care for his own mother.

PERSONAL GROOMING

Brushing Teeth

When: Before breakfast and after dinner

How Often: Twice a day

Technique: During the early stages, your LO will be able to brush their teeth on their own, but they may often forget. Your job is to gently remind them, and then make sure they are doing it correctly. You could help by applying toothpaste to the toothbrush and hand it to your LO, or brush your teeth at the same time so that your LO can mirror your actions.

In the moderate and late stages, you will have to help your LO brush their teeth. In the beginning, stand next to your LO in front of the bathroom sink, if they are about your height. If not, sit down on a chair and have them sit in a chair or on the toilet seat. Then place your hand gently over your LO's hand and guide the toothbrush:

- Use a small, soft-headed toothbrush with a small amount of toothpaste. A smaller brush is easier to get around the back teeth. Remember, swallowing large amounts of toothpaste is a health hazard that can lead to convulsions; diarrhea; difficulty breathing; drooling; and in some instances, a slow heart rate, shock, or heart attack.

- Teeth should be brushed gently using a small circular motion, covering all sides and top. If your LO is firmly gripping the toothbrush they are brushing too hard. Make sure they are angling the toothbrush toward the gumline in order to clean between the gums and teeth.

- Brush the tongue and rinse their mouth when finished.

When you are finished, have your LO swish some water in their mouth and spit it into the sink. If the bathroom is too small for the two of you to sit comfortably and you need to brush their teeth in another room, have them use a plastic basin you can get online: look for an *emesis basin*.

When your LO can no longer brush their teeth, choose a comfortable position where you can see well inside their mouth: sitting or standing to the front, to the side, or behind your LO. Use the same technique at the same time and place every day. First, check between the teeth and cheeks for bits of food, swiping the area with a damp gauze pad. Then use a *soft mouth rest* (like a dentist would use) to help keep your LO's mouth open; it will also prevent accidental biting.

137

Anchor the mouth rest between the upper and lower back teeth and brush their teeth starting on the opposite side of their mouth, following the directions just given.

Another method nurses use involves two toothbrushes. Standing in back of your LO, use the handle of one brush to pull back their cheek, allowing them to rest their teeth on the handle. Then use the second toothbrush to brush their teeth.

If your LO wears dentures, remove them every night and brush them before putting them into a cup of water (ask the dentist if your LO's dentures require cleaning tablets). Rinse and brush the dentures again in the morning before placing them in your LO's mouth. Empty the water in the cup as soon as you remove the dentures in the morning.

Showering

When: I prefer giving a shower in the evenings because it signals that the day is over, and it's relaxing before bedtime. There will be times when your LO needs to shower again in the morning (if they were incontinent overnight).

How Often: Your LO should be bathed every day, no matter what stage they are in. This is helpful for setting up routines, and particularly important for women in order to avoid urinary tract infections.

Technique: In the early stages your LO will likely be able to shower themselves, even though they require help with other ADLs. I once worked with a woman with AD who was in Stage 3. She could shower on her own but couldn't cook for herself. I was hired to provide a daily check-in and prepare meals. Our routine began when I arrived to make dinner. She used the time while I was cooking to take a shower safely, knowing that someone was in the home. This single routine anchored her entire day.

In the early stages your LO can choose between a bath or a shower. However, once they require a full-time caregiver, a bath should no longer be an option. Your LO could easily fall getting in or out of the bathtub, or you can hurt yourself assisting them. The safer choice is showering with a shower chair if they need to sit down.

You will know your LO is no longer capable of showering alone when they cannot follow your directives or are unsteady on their feet at other times during the day. When this happens, lead them to the shower, and if they still seem confused, hand them soap or body wash and a washcloth with a directive to take a shower. Then your LO can shower as you stand outside the bathroom door. Use gentle instructions to make sure that they're soaping up their entire body, washing their hair, and rinsing off properly. In this phase, do not close or lock the door. Have your LO move the soap and shampoo from one side of the shower floor to the other after they have completed the task. It's an easy way for you to check on them.

In the moderate stages you will be washing your LO once you've seen signs that they don't know what to do in the shower. Have them sit on a shower chair and attend to them as you stand outside the shower, using a detachable, handheld shower head. Play soft music to provide a relaxing atmosphere. Use warm water instead of hot, and a milder water pressure instead of full force. Use a washcloth to soap them up, making sure to wash their body completely. Ask them to close their eyes as you shampoo and rinse their hair. They can also hold a washcloth over their eyes for more protection.

By following these instructions to the letter, with practice and putting just a little distance between you and your LO, you're not going to get too wet as you attend to them. At the beginning, you might want to wear a plastic apron to protect yourself and your clothes.

People with dementia/AD often become agitated about the idea of taking a shower. Some become uncomfortable getting their body wet. If they can communicate why they are refusing, you may be able to find a solution, like adding a ceiling heat lamp to a cold bathroom (always keeping safety in mind). If your LO is modest and refuses to undress completely, wash them while they are wearing their underwear/bra, starting with the feet and working up the body. Eventually they will take off their underwear once they have relaxed. If your LO still refuses to get wet, you can experiment with waterless body washes and dry shampoos.

In the later stages, when your LO is less mobile, try a shower-sized wheelchair that doubles as a bedside commode, or switch entirely to a sponge bath. For a sponge bath, have your LO stand or sit on a towel. Fill the bathroom sink with warm, soapy water and a washcloth. Wring out excess water and wash them starting with the face and shoulders, working your way down the body. Then refill the sink with clean water and use another washcloth to rinse off any soapy residue.

If you are going to sponge-bathe your LO in their bed, you will also need two basins: one for soapy water and one for rinsing, and a waterproof cloth to keep the bed dry. You can also purchase an inflatable shampoo basin to make hair washing easier, or switch to dry shampoo.

When your LO is clean, towel them dry. Have them stand up if possible, and if not, have them sit on the toilet lid. Gently pat your LO's skin dry with a towel instead of aggressively rubbing. Make sure that they are completely dry, especially under the breasts and in the groin region, before putting fresh clothes on.

Use body lotion after every shower to prevent dry skin. If you have a television in the bedroom, put the lotion next to the TV remote so that when they turn on the TV, they learn to put the lotion on, too. You can also give them a gentle massage as you apply the lotion all over their body, including hands and feet.

Hair, Skin, and Nails

When/How Often: A good time to attend to all other personal grooming activities is after the shower.

Technique: Keep your LO's nails short so that they don't scratch themselves or you. If your LO is habitually scratching themselves either as a repetitive behavior or because they are uncomfortable, protect their skin by having them wear medical mittens. Another pro tip: if your LO is a man who likes a clean-shaven face, transition them from a manual razor to an electric shaver.

As you're drying off your LO, do a skin assessment. Look for open sores, wounds, cuts, and dry, cracked skin. Gently pinch a fold of skin between your thumb and forefinger on their arm or abdomen. Their skin should quickly return to its original position when released. If it doesn't, your LO may be dehydrated. In Chapter 8, you will learn how to address these issues.

Please Wear Disposable Gloves

Professional caregivers always wear gloves when they perform ADLs with their clients, and you need to wear gloves as well when you are caring for your LO. Every time you bathe, address wounds, or toilet your LO, you are exposing yourself to their body fluids, which may contain germs and cause infections that can spread to you through the skin on your hands. You may also be carrying an infection you don't know about and spread it to your LO. Wearing gloves stops this spread in both directions.

Use a new set of gloves each time you perform an ADL, and immediately throw them away. Then, wash your hands with soap.

GETTING YOUR LO DRESSED
AND EVALUATING THEIR CLOTHING

If you are seeing that your LO is wearing the same clothes every day, it's time for you to take charge of choosing their outfits. Every day, your LO should be dressed in clean clothes in the morning, and undressed and put into clean pajamas for sleeping. In the early stage and the beginning of the moderate stage, it may be helpful to lay out an appropriate outfit on your LO's bed, in the order that the clothes should be put on. If you and your LO will be going out together, wear the same colors in case you are separated so that you remember what they are wearing.

When your LO starts struggling with dressing themselves, reevaluate their closet. Replace items with lots of buttons with comfortable and washable clothes, known to nurses as *adaptive clothing*. These are items that are easier to put on and take off, both for your LO and later, for you. Choose pants with elastic waistbands and snaps (instead of buttons or zippers), and make sure they have lots of pockets (people with dementia love pockets). Tops should have front closures with snaps and zippers rather than buttons: your LO should not be wearing sweaters, sweatshirts, or tops that have to be pulled over the head (no more turtlenecks or crew-necked T-shirts). If your LO is a woman, replace bras with stretchy camisoles or tank tops so that they are supported under their clothes. Look for sundresses that button up the front. Choose sneakers with Velcro closures or loafers: all shoes should have lightweight soles and nonslip rubber bottoms. Using a long-handled shoe horn (at least 12 inches) to help your LO into their shoes will save your back.

In the very last stages of the disease, when your LO is bedridden and showing signs that the end is near, you can make adaptive clothing for them. Take a large T-shirt and cut it straight up the center of the back panel so that they are covered on the front and their clothes are easy to put on and take off. What's more, an open back means that there's less friction between their clothes and the sheets, which provides for easier movement for your LO.

Wearable IDs

I'm a strong advocate for wearable IDs as soon as your LO is diagnosed, especially in the early stages, when they may still be traveling or doing errands on their own. A tracking app that connects your mobile phone to your LO's a a great way to start, but is only effective as long as they continue to carry their phone with them wherever they go. In the moderate stages, it is likely that your LO may wander out of the home or away from you when you are outside. At this point they may also be forgetting to take their phone, and one way to find them quickly is to have them wear an ID bracelet all day.

There are many varieties to choose from: some come with tracking programs, like MedicAlert. An annual fee allows you to report when your LO is missing, and they will contact the local police. The Alzheimer's Association has scholarship money set aside for families to cover this fee.

For simpler options, look for a comfortable rubber or plastic bracelet, or ones where you can change the colors of the straps to match an outfit. A low-tech approach is a wide plastic wristband with locking plastic snaps that you can write on. This one will make sure that your LO can't remove it on their own.

No matter what style, the ID should have your LO's name, address, and diagnosis, as well as your name and telephone number. If your LO has an allergy to a specific medication or food, you can include that information as well.

In the moderate and later stages, you will have to dress your LO. Continue to lay out their outfit on the bed, and announce each time you are picking up an item and helping them into it, as in, *"Now it's time to put on your pants."* Many adaptive clothing items, like pants, sweaters, and shirts, have an opening in the back, which makes dressing easier and puts less pressure on your LO's skin, so that they don't develop bedsores.

At any stage, don't be surprised if your LO complains that they are cold all the time. Older people in general have a hard time maintaining a normal body temperature. Dress them according to how they feel rather than the weather: this may mean adding an extra layer of clothing at all times, and in all seasons. If their hands are very cold, they can even wear mittens or gloves indoors. There are also arm and leg warmers that pull on like socks; these will keep them warm and protect your LO's skin.

Toileting

Toileting is probably the ADL that new caregivers are the most nervous or hesitant about. Like it or not, you need to make sure that your LO is using the bathroom regularly and cleaning themselves correctly afterward.

When/How Often: By the end of the early stages and into the moderate stages you will have to remind your LO that they need to use the bathroom every few hours. These reminders should be built into your Family Care Plan. Toward the end of the moderate stages your LO may start having toileting accidents. This is when you can transition them from washable underwear to disposable underwear. At this point you need to make sure that they are clean and dry so that they don't develop rashes, infections, and, for women, urinary tract infections caused by exposure to fecal matter. The first step in assistance is to place flushable wipes in the bathroom, and remind your LO to use them. In the later stages you will be responsible for cleaning your LO.

Technique: First, always put on a pair of clean medical-grade gloves before you begin toileting. Women need to have their vagina and buttocks wiped from front to back. If your LO is a woman, do not clean her with a shower head after a bowel movement, as this forces microbes into the urethra.

For men, make sure that they are clean under their testicles. No matter who you are caring for, avoid contact with your LO's stool. Use extra toilet tissue and repeat wiping until the paper is clean, and then wash your hands. The elderly have fragile skin, so be especially gentle to prevent skin tears or injury. Never scrub the skin around the anus, which can cause small tears and lead to infection. You can also use flushable wipes, wet toilet paper, or a wet washcloth (which needs to be laundered immediately afterward, along with any soiled clothing).

In Stage 7, when your LO is likely to be bedridden, move to adult diapers with tabs, which are easier for you to put on and take off compared to disposable underwear. Use a protective ointment, the same you would use for a baby, around the rectum, vagina, or penis, every time you change them.

More ADL Items Medicare Covers

- Canes
- Hand-grabber (to pick up items dropped on the ground)
- Home infusion services (for severe dehydration), including pumps and supplies
- Suction pumps
- Traction equipment
- Walkers
- Wheelchairs and scooters

PROVIDING ASSISTANCE WITH WALKING

If your LO needs a walker, cane, or wheelchair, make sure it is the right size. I see lots of people using walkers that are too small for them. The giveaway is that they are leaning or hunched over. There is absolutely no need for this because most walkers are adjustable. To check if it's the appropriate height, have your LO step inside the walker and stand up straight. The top of the walker should line up with the crease on the inside of their wrist. Your LO will not use the walker to help them sit or stand: that's where you come in (see the section on transferring that follows). However, you can walk beside or behind your LO, with your hand on their lower back for support. Let them control the speed that you are both walking, and encourage them to look forward instead of looking down at their feet.

There are several types of walkers: ones that roll, ones that you have to lift to move forward, ones that go directly into the shower, and, my personal favorite, the rollator, which has a basket and a seat in front that doubles as a portable chair. Your LO may need different walkers for each room, or for outdoor and indoor use. One woman I took care of had different-sized walkers in her home. Even though she had recently renovated her apartment, she didn't think about aging in place, and the kitchen and bathroom entranceways were much smaller than the rest. She had to buy one walker for those rooms and a larger one to use in the rest of the apartment. If she had thought about this issue earlier, she could have widened all the doorways during the renovation and only require one walker.

Walkers cannot be used on stairs. If you live in a home with more than one level, rent or buy a stair lift, which is a motorized chair to move your LO up or down a flight of stairs. Or arrange the home so your LO doesn't have to climb stairs: move their bedroom into a den or living room on the main level.

Transferring from Sitting to Standing

The inability to transition on one's own from sitting to standing, or the reverse, typically appears in the moderate stage. The following techniques are critical for protecting both you and your LO. They ensure that your LO doesn't fall, and that you don't injure your back.

If your LO is sitting in a chair and you need them to stand up, let them know that you are going to move them. It's a good idea to hand them something to hold, such as a washcloth or a fidget toy, because when someone's hands are busy, they will be less likely to grab on to you or to the furniture and pull you down. If your LO is strong enough to stand up but weak on one side, have them scoot to the edge of the chair with their feet flat on the floor. Stand by their weak side, legs bent at the knees, and put one hand on their back, facing in the same direction they are going to move, and guide them to a standing position. Then take small steps to move your LO toward their walker or wheelchair.

Another strategy is to stand in front of your LO and ask them to put their arms around your neck. This is a good idea if your LO is weak. Bend at the knees and straighten both of you up by using your thigh muscles, not your back. Place your arms around their waist and lift them to a standing position, holding them as close as possible to avoid straining.

You can also use a Posey or gait belt, which is a strong band used as a transfer tool. They are effective as long as your LO is strong enough to assist you with their legs or arms. When you're not using a gait belt, you can wear it around your waist to keep it handy. Have your LO slide to the edge of the chair or bed if they are able (if they aren't, you will have to switch to a two-person lift; see the instructions that follow). Tell your LO to sit up straight with their feet slightly apart so that you can get one foot in between their feet for leverage. Use the leg that corresponds to the direction you will be going; if you are moving to the left, use your left leg. Your LO should put their hands on your forearms, not around your neck. Wrap the belt around your LO's waist and tighten it just enough so that you can get your fingers between your LO and the belt. Face your LO and pull them up by putting your hands on the back of the belt. Bend your knees and lift up.

You can also use real, medical-grade tools that you are entitled to. A power chair that goes from sitting to standing will guide your LO upright or provide a place for them to lie completely vertically to take a nap without moving them into the bed. When they can no longer walk on their own, a hydraulic manual lift offers a safe way to move your LO out of a bed or chair.

The Two-Person Transfer

You may not be able to transition your LO alone. If this is the case, alter your Family Care Plan so that there is an extra pair of hands available at the right times of day. For example, have a team member come over in the morning so that you can transfer your LO out of bed and into another room for breakfast and grooming. The team member then stays for an hour or two (at most) while you run errands. When you return, your LO will be ready to be transferred again. For a two-person transfer, your LO should be seated with each person standing at their left and right sides. Your LO puts their arms around the two caregivers' backs, and you and your team member each put an arm around the LO's back, under their arms. Bending down, each person uses their free hand to reach under the LO's legs. On the count of three, each caregiver lifts the LO straight up, using their legs and keeping a strong back. Then walk your LO to the new location and lower them gently into place.

Transferring from Lying Down to Standing

In the moderate stages, your LO may need help getting out of bed. Have your LO sit up straight. If they cannot pivot, use the handles of the cotton pad on top of the draw sheet to swing your LO to where their legs are hanging over the side of the bed. Use the transfer method that is most comfortable for you to get them to a standing position.

In the late stages, you will need to help your LO out of bed and into a wheelchair. First, place the wheelchair as close to your LO as possible. If they are able, have your LO sit up. If they are not, they should be transitioned into a hospital bed as quickly as possible. Otherwise, getting your LO out of bed will require a two-person transfer.

From a hospital bed, elevate the head of the bed until your LO is in a sitting position. Use the handles of the cotton pad sitting on top of the draw sheet to swing your LO until their legs are hanging over the side of the bed. Use the transfer method that is most comfortable for you to place your LO into the wheelchair. Lastly, unlock the wheels and move away from the bed.

Basic Rules for a Wheelchair Transfer

Every time you transfer your LO into a wheelchair, lock the wheels and keep them locked until your LO is comfortably seated. The foot pedals and/or leg rests should be moved out of the way.

Once you're ready to move, gently guide the wheelchair forward. If you are going up a curb or stairs, pull the wheelchair backward; before you do so, place a Posey belt around your LO's waist and the back of the chair to secure them.

CHAPTER 6

Filling the Family Care Plan
with Appropriate Activities

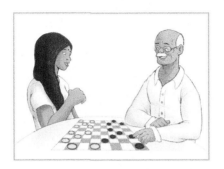

Caregiving can be tedious when every day looks like the one before and the one yet to come. That's why professional nurses like me rely on a care plan: it is the best tool for structuring your day and preventing burnout. Your Family Care Plan takes the guesswork out of caregiving and puts you in a proactive mode as opposed to a reactive one. As I've said before, planning ahead is being proactive and is the key to lowering your daily stress so that you can provide exceptional care.

Nursing homes, SNIFs, and memory care units are highly scheduled to help the caregivers, and I think this model works. The Family Care Plan lets you put together an engaging schedule that you can stick with and develop routines that are individualized and mentally/physically engaging, creating a holistic approach to daily living.

My care plans are typically set for two weeks at a time. This allows for enough planning and enough flexibility if I need to make changes.

As you learned in Chapter 2, a Family Care Plan for someone in the early stages is a rough outline of the day. As the disease progresses, these schedules will become more detailed and take an hour-by-hour approach. By the late stages, you may have to break up hourlong activities into 15-to-30-minute intervals and build in reminders for you to attend to your LO's toileting needs and snacks between meals.

ACTIVITIES ARE THE BACKBONE OF A GOOD FAMILY CARE PLAN

With the ADLs out of the way, it's time to make the most of the rest of the day with your LO. I fill each day with activities that appropriately match my patient's interests as well as their mental and physical abilities. An activity doesn't have to cost much, be complicated or messy, or take place outside the home. Using the broadest definition possible, an activity is any way you decide to spend your time that is purposeful and meaningful.

Activities can include old hobbies or new interests, entertainment, housework, and self-care. A good activity may be sitting on the porch and watching the birds for an hour in the late afternoon, or tackling a new craft like clay. It can also be an adult daycare visit, dinner at a restaurant, or a walk in the park. No matter what you choose, activities should on some level help your LO maintain skills or provide exercise and mental stimulation. Watching television for hours on end alone is not an activity, but watching a movie with someone else counts.

Incorporating a variety of daily activities can elevate your LO's overall mood. Any opportunity to focus on something creative or an activity that provides mental or physical stimulation will enhance their quality of life, distract from negative feelings, and reduce agitation. These benefits linger throughout the day, not only when your LO is engaged in the activity. Keep in mind that organizing or participating in an activity should not increase your stress level or your LO's. Instead, it should alleviate stress by allowing your LO to maintain some semblance of independence and a sense of self-worth, self-esteem, and inclusion. For you, activities provide an opportunity to connect with your LO and a creative or physical outlet for yourself.

Meet Mel

My neighbor Mel has dementia. I often see him in the afternoons sitting on his porch, talking to a baseball coach and a few of the boys on his team. Mel's wife, Anna, told me that Mel has always loved baseball, and whenever he hears the young men playing on the field, he gets up and goes to the window. Dave, the coach, noticed Mel watching one day and realized that Mel needed to socialize. He set up a routine with Anna for Mel, and every day he brings over a couple of boys for an hour after practice and they all talk together. Anna told me that this 1-hour routine has become the highlight of Mel's day: he lights up as he puts on his coat to go outside to spend time with the kids.

Anna also confided that before this arrangement, Mel was lonely. Loneliness is not a good thing when you have dementia, and it can set in even when you are spending the whole day with your LO. This tiny activity accomplishes so much for Mel: he gets to be outside in the fresh air and socialize with other people, and he has something to look forward to that anchors his day.

WHEN TO SCHEDULE ACTIVITIES

The "when" of scheduling activities is just as important as choosing which to try. I find that the best time to start an activity is when the person with dementia/AD has the most energy, because that's when they are able to stay focused. Some people with dementia are raring to go first thing, or right after breakfast, or after an afternoon nap. Others are their best selves later in the day. For instance, my aunt liked to stay up late watching sports and was a late sleeper. We started her day around 10:00 a.m. Once she was up, she was fine for the rest of the day and could do an activity or two without getting too tired.

As you get to know your LO better, you will be able to gauge when they are ready to try an activity. You want to provide enough stimulation to keep them engaged during the activity and somewhat tired afterward. At the same time, you don't want to plan too much in one day, which can lead to frustration or agitation. You also have to get a sense of their environment, including their neighborhood. You'll want to know what time the closest park closes, or if the streets are well-lit for an evening stroll. Is there a nice place to be outside within walking distance from home, or will you have to use a car or public transportation? Is there a particular destination they like to visit? All of this information can also help structure your day and influence which activities you plan for.

Activities should be closely monitored, as your LO's abilities will decline as their dementia progresses. In the earlier stages, you may be able to set your LO up with an activity, like a craft, while you prepare dinner. This could be a nice routine for a while, until one day you find that it no longer works at all. If you're flexible, and you're expecting change (because you're not in denial), you'll be able to quickly adjust the activity to one that you can do together at another time during the day, or swap it out for a different activity.

Your LO will experience a range of emotions throughout one day, and certain activities may trigger these emotional shifts. For instance, at the end of the day, people with dementia/AD often get despondent, which is a pattern called *sundowning* that we will discuss more in the next chapter. During this time, they become agitated; it is not the right moment to start an activity.

If you see that your LO is getting restless and doesn't want to participate any longer in any particular activity, don't force it on them. All that will accomplish is making them more upset. Instead, have a backup activity at the ready that meets the same goal and redirect them toward it.

CAPABILITY FACTORS TO KEEP IN MIND

A person's intellectual and physical abilities can fluctuate within the stages of dementia because of another illness, stress, fatigue, or mood. This change in function may be permanent or temporary depending on the cause. What's more, your LO will have good days when they are cooperative and engaged, and bad days when they may feel like being left alone.

When an activity doesn't seem to work for your LO, it doesn't mean that you have to put it away forever. You can try it again at another time, or when these other factors may not be in play. If you try it again and it's still a bust, it's possible that your LO has permanently lost the ability to participate in that particular task.

Your LO's competence is also influenced by emotional, physical, and cognitive factors. Your LO may be able to do a particular activity, but if the motivation does not exist, they will not seem capable. Once their motivation increases, it may appear that they have "learned" a skill. However, the skill was there all along. Still, take it as a compliment that you've increased their motivation enough so that they share their ability with you.

Lastly, keep your LO's attention span in mind. Early-stage activities can last an entire morning or afternoon. In the moderate stages, keep them to about 1 hour; if the activity is a game, you may be able to play more than once, or two different games. If your LO is in the moderate stages, one indoor and one outdoor activity per day is probably all that they can manage. In the late stages, activities should be thought of in 15-to-20-minute increments: one game. The number of activities you will be able to do in one day will be entirely determined by their daytime sleeping schedule.

In general, these guidelines match stages and capabilities:

Early stages: Choose activities that focus on the whole task: reading a book or listening to an audiobook/podcast, sculpting with clay, drawing, or coloring.

Mid-stages: Choose activities that focus on individual steps: a board game or organizing a photo album.

Late stages: Choose activities that focus on the senses (hearing, touch, taste, smell, movement, and vision): listening to music or rummaging through a sensory box.

ACTIVITIES TO MAINTAIN REGULAR LIFE

Many activities can keep your LO engaged in their old life. Your job as a caregiver is to help them participate in these activities for as long as possible, and then modify them as they move from one stage to another. At the same time, you don't want to put your LO, or yourself, in a dangerous situation, or one that feels increasingly burdensome. Just because your LO used to love clothes shopping, if that outing is too stressful for you, it's no longer a good fit. Modify their hobby by setting aside an hour a week to look at catalogs or magazines together, or browse the Internet for their favorite items.

Give gentle reminders for these daily tasks, and just because your LO won't remember what to do, it doesn't mean that they can't do it. My aunt was walking well until she passed, and was physically fit to do most daily tasks on her own, but she needed to be reminded *how* to do them every time.

Work the following tasks into your weekly care plan:

BASIC HOUSEKEEPING

In the early stages, your LO may get a sense of accomplishment from tidying up more than games or events, because such tasks are purposeful and allow them to maintain a sense of contribution. The following suggestions are safe activities for people in the early and moderate stages, but remember: everyone is different. And no matter what stage they are in, you need to be around to supervise, or even participate:

Laundry: Well into the moderate stages, your LO can help you sort and fold clean clothes. However, you should be the one to put them away because your LO may not remember where everything goes and may stash them in the wrong places.

Mopping/sweeping/vacuuming: Taking care of floors is an ideal task for someone with dementia because there is little that can be inadvertently broken. However, the noise of the vacuum cleaner may not work for some people. Vacuuming can be either very soothing or very agitating.

Making the bed: This is another good option for a daily low-risk-for-injury task. Ask your LO how they like their bed made and follow their lead; some people like their sheets tightly tucked in, while others prefer a looser bed.

Managing their collections: People with dementia/AD love to collect things, and an activity can be organizing and storing the stuff they've acquired over the years.

Putting dishes away: This activity is appropriate with supervision, as long as you've switched to non-breakable dishware.

GROCERY SHOPPING

In the early stages, grocery shopping is a safe activity to do together. I recommend that you go with your LO, even if they are able to drive and carry items into the home. The supermarket can be overwhelming, and they may not buy what they need or what is on their shopping list. Instead, they may overbuy or underbuy, which means that you will have to take a second trip to the store. However, the experience is good for both socialization and exercise.

Try going to the grocery store when it is likely to be less crowded. When this activity no longer suits you or your LO, switch it up: you do the food shopping and then have your LO help you put away the groceries, while you watch.

ACTIVITIES IN THE HOME

Build your list of activities based on how your LO already enjoys spending time. In the early stages your LO will be able to share what they love to do (if you don't know already), and it's a good idea to make a list with them of things they would like to continue doing, or try for the first time. This list can include hobbies, games, types of exercise, opportunities for socialization, religious services or groups, creative arts outlets, and more. As your LO moves into the moderate and later stages and has difficulty communicating, this list will provide a guideline.

Your LO will want to participate in the activities they've always enjoyed until they no longer have the ability, and then those activities become frustrating. Your job is to make activities meaningful and easy: to let them do the things they want to do for as long as possible. Then, when they can't, introduce new things that are equally stimulating and fun. Don't hesitate to introduce activities that you like, too. Often, people think they won't enjoy something because they believe it's not available to them or they are not entitled to it, like listening to opera. Or they had never been exposed to it, like going to a museum.

If possible, keep activities relegated to one area of the home, like the living room or den. This will help your LO frame activities with a beginning and end when you move into this space. Leaving visual cues out, such as placing a deck of cards on the coffee table, lets your LO know what to expect and can create additional opportunities to play. Stay positive when you engage in any pastime, and give the power to your LO so that you can go through it at their pace. You may have to modify the rules of the game to meet their competency. If you are playing a game or working on art or a craft, break it down into simple steps and say what you are going to do before you do it.

The following lists are suggestions that are geared to specific stages. All of them are geared to be enjoyable for you both. They are also meant to enhance your LO's cognitive skills, provide opportunities for learning and socialization, and improve mood.

ARTS AND CRAFTS

Art projects are cathartic for both you and your LO, as they allow us to express the thoughts and emotions that can be tough to say out loud. This is particularly helpful when your LO is struggling with finding the right words. For you, art can be an outlet for expressing emotions you may not feel comfortable sharing. Art also provides creative stimulation and helps your LO maintain fine motor skills; this is critical for maintaining the competencies needed for the ADLs, like dressing and bathing. Creating art also increases confidence, concentration, and motivation. Best of all, it is an activity that you and your LO can do together in a parallel manner: at the same time, but not always involved in each other's project. My friend Carla is an illustrator who is taking care of her mother, and they paint together every day for an hour. Her mother loves that they are doing a creative activity together, and Carla loves that she can teach her mother a new skill.

I believe that all arts and crafts are appropriate for people with dementia/AD with the right supervision. I have found that this group of people particularly enjoy arts and crafts that involve repetitive motions. Here are some of my favorite suggestions:

- Clay or moldable crafts, like pipe cleaners

- Coloring books: LOs in the early stages can use adult coloring books with intricate designs and patterns. As the disease progresses, move on to children's coloring books, and eventually blank sheets of paper.

- Creating collages (with images already cut for moderate and late stages)

- Drawing/painting: As the disease progresses, your LO's fine motor skills will diminish, even if they were an accomplished artist in the past. Provide materials that meet their abilities. You may move from colored pencils to finger paints, or fine brushes to wide brushes as they move from one stage to another. Paint-by-number projects come in a variety of skill levels.

- Journaling/creative writing: Any writing prompts are appropriate for the early stages. As they move to the moderate stages, they can journal by making photo albums, collages, or other types of original artwork. If your LO likes to tell stories but is having difficulty writing as they move into the moderate stages, you can literally turn their stories into an oral history by recording them speaking their stories (use the voice memo feature on your phone). Or you can record the stories and have them transcribed into a document you can keep.

- Lego or other connecting blocks: Your LO can either follow the instructions to put the sets together, or connect the pieces to make their own creations. As the disease progresses, move on to sets with fewer and larger pieces.

- Making photo albums: Create one of just you and your LO that chronicles your time together.

- Puzzles: LOs in the early stages can try adult puzzles with clear images. As the disease progresses, move on to children's puzzles, with fewer and larger pieces.

- Sewing projects like needlepoint, knitting, crochet, or quilting: These activities need to be carefully monitored because your LO will be using a needle.

During any arts and crafts, limit choices to one or two: one or two colors, mediums, or tools. Sit near your LO and participate in the activity with them. As their disease progresses, modify the activity (if they enjoy it, and if they don't substitute another one) with larger tools or fewer pieces. Your LO may need a visual demonstration to get them started, and as I've said earlier, they may need this cue each time you start the activity. I often provide "hand-over-hand" assistance to initiate the action or movement in the moderate and late stages. Lastly, go easy with your expectations. Your LO is not going to magically produce museum-quality work. It is unlikely that they will recognize errors, and there's no point in correcting anything unless your LO demonstrates frustration with the project.

BOARD GAMES

If your LO was always a game player, start with the games they are familiar with. It's amazing to see that even when the disease progresses and they lose the ability to recall names, they will remember the rules of complex games. It's a pleasure to watch your LO play and win!

When your LO can no longer play the games they loved, choose easier versions of similar pastimes. For example, if they loved chess, try checkers using the pieces from their chess set to keep them engaged. Even in the early stages, though, I don't recommend word games, games with a time limit, or games that make loud noises: all may cause frustration and reduce self-confidence.

The games I recommend for the early stages include the following:

- Backgammon
- Chess
- Chinese checkers
- Pictionary
- Rummikub
- Sequence for Adults

The games I recommend for the moderate stages and the beginning of the late stages include the following:

- Candy Land
- Checkers
- Connect 4

- Dominoes
- Guess Who?
- Hedbanz
- Life on Earth
- Lotería (Mexican bingo)
- Ludo
- Parcheesi
- Pokeno
- Qwirkle
- Sequence for Children
- Sorry!

CARD GAMES

Like board games, if your LO was always a card player, start with the games they love. Again, even when the disease progresses and they lose the ability to recall names, they will remember the rules of complex games. It's a pleasure to watch your LO play—and win! What's more, card games are social in nature; the longer that you facilitate a regular game with their friends, the better.

In the early stages, your LO can master a variety of card games. As the disease progresses, card games that are geared to children, like UNO, Go Fish, and Old Maid, will be appropriately challenging.

CONVERSATION

Creating moments of engagement between you and your LO that are outside the ADLs or meals can be an activity in and of itself.

Recounting family history and personal stories or even sharing thoughts about a book or a movie kick-starts the brain into action. What's more, it may let you see an entirely new side of your LO as you learn about their preferences, hopes, and memories, and unearthing pleasant reminders of the past may help your LO feel more stable and confident.

A conversation scheduled into every day, or even weekly, is an ideal way to spend an hour. You and your LO can take turns starting the conversation with a topic of your choosing. As time passes, you may feel like you've explored every subject under the sun. That's when conversation cards come in handy; these are decks of cards that have conversation starters printed on them. You can pick a card randomly and explore a whole new topic. You could also try aromatherapy; stimulating any of the five senses can bring up memories, and smells are particularly effective. You don't have to buy a bunch of essential oils; have your LO smell foods, unlit scented candles, or perfumes, and see what positive memories they evoke.

No matter how you start a conversation, keep it going. I'm a naturally curious person, so when I chat with anyone, I ask a lot of questions. I've honed my technique based on the greatest-of-all-time interviewers: Larry King and Oprah. King had a specific style I find works well with people with dementia/AD, which revolves around one rule: listen to the answer, because the answer can often lead to the next question. This technique helps to keep the conversation going, and if you are open, you may learn something new. Oprah, meanwhile, is especially kind when asking questions; she doesn't make people feel uncomfortable. At the same time, she's direct, which leads to people giving their most honest answer.

I learned a lot about my aunt's upbringing only by asking questions, listening to the answers, and then asking follow-ups. It gave me an entirely fresh perspective on my own family. I also learned that my aunt was able to retain an enormous amount of information regarding sports. When she was in the moderate stages and seemed like she couldn't remember anything, she could tell you all about LeBron James, his most recent game, how much money he had (and what good things he was doing with it), and how his season was going. She also closely followed the New York Mets.

MUSIC

I can't stress enough the importance of music for people with dementia/AD. In fact, I've seen firsthand how music therapy in nursing homes can transform a nonverbal patient into a singing wonder. It is nothing short of miraculous.

Researchers have found that musical memories are preserved in those with dementia/AD because the areas in the brain that store them are relatively undamaged by the disease. A person with dementia/AD is able to recall their oldest memories far longer than more recent ones. Even as they lose the ability to remember what has happened as far back as a decade or two, they retain the memories of their childhood until the end. This means that if you want to use music as an activity (or even keep it playing in the background to relieve stress, anxiety, and agitation), choose your LO's cherished music from their childhood or what is known as "the courting years" of their teens and twenties. Other research has found that new songs help forge new memories. You can try to introduce your LO to the music that you like, and see how they respond. They may be able to memorize the song and sing along, or relate it to another activity.

Set up a sing-along or a "name that tune" game, or match movement to music with dance or a restorative yoga practice. Or play new and old songs as a departure point for discussion or reminiscence. Watch your LO's responses carefully: If they enjoy a song, keep going. If they have a negative reaction, take it off your playlist.

READING

People in the early stages of dementia/AD can still read, and many love to do so. It's an activity that really fills the day. However, there will be a point where it becomes difficult to keep track of the characters or storyline in a book. When this happens, I have my early-stage patients read a book while listening to the audiobook version at the same time. They still have the experience of holding the book and turning the pages, without the frustration of losing their place or forgetting what they just read and having to start over.

As the disease progresses, I switch to simpler books. One activity I've found to be particularly entertaining for my patients with moderate- and late-stage dementia/AD is reintroducing children's books that I read aloud to them. It's an activity that reignites memories of beloved books. It also sparks interesting conversations.

Or switch entirely to audiobooks. Play an audiobook over a smart speaker so that your LO doesn't have to sit with headphones, which can be uncomfortable. You can buy audiobooks or borrow them from your local library.

> ### Learn Something New Together
>
> A fun activity is to learn about a new place or hobby, and then take that knowledge into an experiential dimension. You and your LO can read books, watch movies, or research a country you've never visited. Cook foods from that country, create art that represents what you've learned, or try a craft from that country for a tactile experience. You can imagine what it would be like to go there, talk about it as an activity, and even pack a real suitcase.

RUMMAGE/SENSORY BOXES AND FIDGET TOYS/BLANKETS

People with dementia/AD find it soothing to keep something in their hands. These boxes, blankets, and toys allow your LO to feel a variety of textures and to explore items with an open sense of curiosity. In essence, you are bringing the world to them. These tools are very effective, especially in the moderate and late stages.

You can purchase these products or make your own. Collect a variety of textures—that aren't sharp—and place them in a box or sew them onto a blanket. Include yarn, fabrics, beaded necklaces, fur, coins, shells, buttons, cubes, and so on. Your LO can touch them whenever they get agitated (see Chapter 7). As another sensory activity, have them see if they can identify the object without looking at it.

TELEVISION

Television can be the greatest babysitter of all time, but sticking your LO in front of it is not an activity. Don't get me wrong: there will be a time, probably daily, when you will thank the creators of television and on-demand streaming services. I'm not saying that your LO shouldn't watch the shows they love; just don't count it as an activity.

Some of my clients are so deeply engaged with their shows that they are calmer when they are watching them. It counts as an activity if you watch *with* your LO and discuss what you are seeing before, during, and afterward. Movies count. So do game shows: my patients are wild for *Wheel of Fortune*, *The Price Is Right*, *To Tell the Truth*, *Family Feud*, and *Let's Make a Deal*. I'm not sure if it's the lighting or the excitement from the crowd that's contagious, but a good game show often improves my patients' mood. I've seen people with dementia/AD respond well to competition shows like *The Masked Singer* or *America's Got Talent* as well. Many streaming services and cable television providers carry the Game Show Network, which is exactly as it sounds: 24/7 game shows!

End the Day with a Relaxing Activity

Between dinner and bedtime, a brief activity like listening to calming music or a meditation (see Chapter 3) signals that the day is winding down and ends the day on a positive note. Limiting exposure to bright lights will help your LO get a better night's sleep, so don't spend the evening watching television or using a computer or smartphone.

DAILY PHYSICAL ACTIVITY

One of the most profound impacts of exercise on your LO is improving their independence in the early and moderate stages. Just as doing crafts enhances fine motor skills, strength exercises protect muscles from atrophy, and cardio/aerobics enhance endurance during the day and improve sleep at night. Exercise also improves blood flow in the brain, which keeps it active and may even slow the progression of dementia/AD. Exercise boosts mood and self-confidence and is an excellent antidote for depression and anxiety, possibly even more than antidepressants.[1] If nothing else, if your LO feels physically fit and capable, they will feel better about themselves.

I prescribe 30 minutes per day of aerobic exercise at a moderate exertion. In the early stages, your LO can continue with exercises like tennis or swimming. However, as the disease progresses these activities may no longer be safe, so I suggest switching to taking long walks. Walk outdoors, weather permitting, and at the speed that works best for your LO. This may mean that it is not a real workout for you, and you will have to find another time during the day to get your own exercise in (see Chapter 3).

THE POWER OF WALKING

Taking a walk has so many positives: it provides a much-needed change of scenery, exercise, connection with the community, and an immersive sensory activity. I recommend what some call an "awe walk" or "walking with wonder." Consciously looking at, listening to, smelling, and touching the small wonders in our world is thought to improve mood, making people feel more hopeful and upbeat.[2] Best of all, an awe walk doesn't have to be far away or in a particular location. While it's nice to mix up your destination from time to time and include a botanical garden or a museum, you and your LO can take an awe walk right outside your home. You can pick a theme before you go out the door, as in *"Let's look for new spring flowers,"* or *"Let's listen for birds."* Or be open to being surprised: once I was taking an awe walk with a client and we came across a pond that was full of frogs. We couldn't see them, but we could hear them!

15 MINUTES OF AMPLIFIED WALKING

If your LO is physically able, chart a 15-minute circuit outside to use for cardio, following Nikki's suggestions below. *Tempo* means going at your regular pace. *Brisk* means taking it up a notch and pumping your arms with each step, in coordination with the opposite leg. If you're having fun and feel like pushing it a little more, do the circuit twice.

- Tempo walk—2 minutes
- Brisk walk—1 minute
- Tempo walk—1 minute
- Brisk walk—2 minutes
- Tempo walk—1 minute
- Brisk walk—3 minute
- Tempo walk—1 minute
- Brisk walk—2 minutes
- Tempo walk—1 minute
- Cool-down (take it even slower)—1 minute

GET YOUR LO FIT WITH NIK

Nikki Kimbrough developed the following safe program with your LO in mind. The goal is to give your LO the best opportunity to continue to meet their own needs by supporting their ability to get up and out of bed, walk around without pain, dress themselves, bend gracefully and pick up things off the ground, reach for things that are stored in high places, and carry a reasonable load.

The following exercises provide a full-body workout that hits all the major muscle groups and raises heart rate. Have your LO do the exercises standing for as long as they can, as it offers a better workout, but the exercises can be completed while sitting in a chair as well. Your LO can go through the entire routine or break up the circuits for a shorter workout; make sure they do the warm-up and cool-down each time.

This workout includes compound movements that work both the upper body and lower body at the same time, which supports cognitive function. Basically, it's the perfect 30-minute mind-body routine. A video with Nikki going through this entire workout is available for you at www.getfitwithnik.com/caregiving-with-love-joy.

WARM-UP
- Inhale/Exhale
- Neck Tilts Side to Side—5x Each Side (10 Total)
- Neck Tilts Chin Down to Chin Up—5x Each Side (10 Total)
- Chicken Neck Chin Forward to Chin Back—5x Each Side (10 Total)
- Neck Isolations Turn Right to Left—5x Each Side (10 Total)
- Neck Circles Right to Left—5x Each Side (10 Total)
- Shoulder Shrugs—5x

- Shoulder Circles Forward and Backward—5x Each Side (10 Total)
- Back Flexion/Extension—5x Each Side (10 Total)
- Alt Side Bends—5x Each Side (10 Total)
- Knee Lifts—5x Each Leg (10 Total)

CIRCUIT I

- Touch and Go (Chair Squats)—10x
- Reach and Pull—10x Each Side
- Jab-Cross Punch Outs—10x Each
- Abductor/Adductor Foot Taps Out-Out-In-In—10x
- Chair Jacks—10x
- Jab-Cross Punch Outs—10x Each
- Single-Leg Leg Extension (Right)—10x
- Single-Leg Leg Extension (Left)—10x
- Jab-Cross Punch Outs—10x Each

CIRCUIT 2

- Double-Leg Extensions—10x
- Chair Jacks with Arnold Pec Deck Back Squeeze—10x
- Chair March Runs—10x Each Leg
- Bicep Arm Curls—10x
- Rotate Wrist and Press—10x
- Chair March Runs—10x Each Leg
- Seated Row—10x
- Triceps Kickbacks—10x
- Chair March Runs—10x Each Leg

CIRCUIT 3

- Ankle (Shin) Hinge Overs—10x
- Single-Arm Rotational Upward Punch (Right Side)—10x

- Seated Crunch—10x
- Ankle (Shin) Hinge Overs to Hammer Curl—10x
- Single-Arm Rotational Upward Punch (Left Side)—10x
- Seated Crunch Pulse—10x
- Ankle (Shin) Hinge Overs to Hammer Curl to Press—10x
- Alternating Rotational Upward Punches (Right to Left)—10x Each Side
- Seated Crunch X10 to Seated Crunch Pulse—10x

CIRCUIT 4
- Clasp Overhead Triceps—10x
- Single-Side Russian Twist (Right)—10x
- Chair Jacks—10x
- Lateral Raise to Front Raise—10x Each
- Single-Side Russian Twist (Left)—10x
- Chair March Runs—10x
- Lateral Raise to Front Raise to Back Squeeze—10x Each
- Double-Side Russian Twist (Left to Right)—10x Each Side
- Touch and Go—10x

COOL-DOWN
- Inhale/Exhale
- Hinge Over toward Ankles to Roll-Ups
- Shoulder Circles Backward and Forward
- Seated Hamstring Stretch (Right to Left)
- Bring Knee into Chest (Right to Left)
- Alt Side Bends—5x Each Side
- Back Flexion/Extension—5x Each Side
- Triceps Stretch to Upper Back Stretch (Right to Left)
- Shoulder Shrugs—5x
- Neck Circles Right to Left—5x Each Side

- Neck Isolations Turn Right to Left—5x Each Side
- Chicken Neck Chin Forward to Chin Back—5x Each Side
- Neck Tilts Chin Down to Chin Up—5x Each Side
- Neck Tilts Side to Side—5x Each Side

Exercise Descriptions/Instructions

WARM-UP

INHALE/EXHALE

- Stand up or sit at the edge of a chair. Your feet should be shoulder width apart, arms by your sides, head straight and looking forward.
- Raise your arms above your head and take in a deep breath.
- Then lower your arms back to your sides and let out your breath.

NECK TILTS SIDE TO SIDE

- Stand up or sit at the edge of a chair. Your feet should be shoulder width apart, arms by your sides, head straight and looking forward.
- Gently tilt your head to the right side, with your right ear toward your shoulder.
- Then gently tilt your head to the left side, with your left ear toward your shoulder.
- Return to center and repeat.

NECK TILTS CHIN DOWN TO CHIN UP

- Stand up or sit at the edge of a chair. Your feet should be shoulder width apart, arms by your sides, head straight and looking forward.

- Gently tilt your head down, with chin tucked in toward your chest.
- Then gently tilt your head back with your chin pointed up.
- Return to center and repeat.

CHICKEN NECK CHIN FORWARD TO CHIN BACK
- Stand up or sit at the edge of a chair. Your feet should be shoulder width apart, arms by your sides, head straight and looking forward.
- Gently protrude your head and chin forward.
- Then gently move your head and chin to the starting point.
- Repeat.

NECK ISOLATIONS TURN RIGHT TO LEFT
- Stand up or sit at the edge of a chair. Your feet should be shoulder width apart, arms by your sides, head straight and looking forward.
- Gently turn your head to the right.
- The gently turn your head to the left.
- Return your head to center and repeat.

NECK CIRCLES
- Stand up or sit at the edge of a chair. Your feet should be shoulder width apart, arms by your sides, head straight and looking forward.
- Gently tilt your head to the right and start rolling back.
- Keep rolling your head to the left and then down.
- Bring your head up to the starting position and repeat in the opposite direction.

SHOULDER SHRUGS

- Stand up or sit at the edge of a chair. Your feet should be shoulder width apart, arms by your sides, head straight and looking forward.
- Raise your shoulders up toward your neck and ears; hold for 2 seconds.
- Then release and repeat.

SHOULDER CIRCLES FORWARD AND BACKWARD

- Stand up or sit at the edge of a chair. Your feet should be shoulder width apart, arms by your sides, head straight and looking forward.
- Slowly rotate your shoulders forward, making big circles.
- Repeat the movement backward until the set is complete.

BACK FLEXION/EXTENSION

- Stand up or sit at the edge of a chair. Your feet should be shoulder width apart, head straight and looking forward, palms facing up.
- Roll your shoulders forward and bend your upper back forward like they are caving in.
- Then return to the starting position and roll your shoulders back, squeezing your shoulder blades. Repeat.

ALT SIDE BENDS

- Stand up or sit at the edge of a chair. Your feet should be shoulder width apart, head straight and looking forward, palms facing up.
- Hinge over to the right side as far as you can, keeping your spine, head and neck in alignment.

- Then come up to the starting position.
- Switch sides.

KNEE LIFTS
- Stand up or sit at the edge of a chair. Your feet should be shoulder width apart, arms by your sides, head straight and looking forward.
- Lift your knee toward the ceiling, hold for 1 to 2 seconds, and return your foot to the floor.
- Then switch sides.

CIRCUIT 1

TOUCH AND GO (CHAIR SQUATS)
- Sit at the edge of a chair with your feet shoulder width apart and your arms by your sides.
- Drive your heels and the middle of your feet down into the ground as you stand up tall. Be sure to keep your chest upright.
- Lower into a squat position by bending at your hips, pushing your hips backward, and bending your knees until you have sat back down in the chair.
- Repeat.

REACH AND PULL
- Stand up or sit at the edge of a chair. Your feet should be shoulder width apart, arms by your sides, head straight and looking forward.
- Breathe deeply as you drive your right knee up toward the ceiling while pulling your hands down and your elbows toward the sides of your waist (chair).

- Return your right foot to the floor while reaching overhead again.
- Switch sides by driving your left knee toward the ceiling while pulling your arms down, then returning your left foot to the floor and reaching overhead.
- Repeat.

JAB-CROSS PUNCH OUTS

- Stand up or sit at the edge of a chair. Your feet should be shoulder width apart, arms by your sides, head straight and looking forward.
- Make fists with your hands and place your arms bent in front of you, with fists about chin level.
- Squeeze your shoulder blades together and engage your abs.
- Then throw quick forward punches, alternating between your left and right arm.
- Repeat.

ABDUCTOR/ADDUCTOR FOOT TAPS OUT-OUT-IN-IN

- Sit at the edge of a chair with your feet shoulder width apart and your hands holding on to the sides of the chair.
- Place your right foot out farther than shoulder width, then place your left foot out farther than shoulder width.
- Bring your right foot back to shoulder width, then bring your left foot back to shoulder width.
- Repeat.

CHAIR JACKS

- Sit at the edge of a chair with your back straight, abs engaged, shoulders relaxed, arms at your sides, and feet together.

- Extend both arms overhead, stepping both legs and feet out to the sides.
- Return both arms to your sides, stepping both legs and feet together.
- Repeat.

SINGLE-LEG LEG EXTENSION (RIGHT AND LEFT)
- Stand up or sit at the edge of a chair. Your feet should be shoulder width apart, arms by your sides, head straight and looking forward.
- Keep your upper body still while you extend and straighten your right leg, then flex your quadriceps muscles. Hold for 1 to 3 seconds before returning to the start position.
- Repeat, then switch sides.

CIRCUIT 2

DOUBLE-LEG EXTENSIONS
- Stand up or sit at the edge of a chair. Your feet should be shoulder width apart, arms by your sides, head straight and looking forward.
- Keep your upper body still while you extend and straighten both legs, then flex your quadriceps muscles. Hold for 1 to 3 seconds before returning to the start position.
- Repeat.

CHAIR JACKS WITH ARNOLD PEC DECK BACK SQUEEZE
- Sit at the edge of a chair, feet on the floor, with feet shoulder width apart.

- Bring your arms up, flexed at shoulder height, closed in toward your chest, with your hands in fists, level with your temples, facing each other.
- Open your arms wide with your fists facing out and aligned with your ears. At the same time, gently squeeze your shoulder blades together for 2 seconds, engaging your back.
- Return your arms to the starting position.
- Repeat.

CHAIR MARCH RUNS
- Sit at the edge of a chair, with your back straight, feet on the floor, arms at your sides.
- Begin by marching with alternate legs. Bring one thigh up as high as possible and return to the starting position, then do the same with your other leg.
- Simultaneously, pump your arms like you are running.

BICEP ARM CURLS
- Stand up or sit at the edge of a chair. Your feet should be shoulder width apart, arms by your sides, head straight and looking forward.
- Put your hands in fist position, fists facing up.
- Keeping your upper arms stable and shoulders relaxed, bend at the elbow and bring your fists toward your shoulders. Your elbows should stay tucked in close to your ribs.
- Then lower your fists to the starting position.
- Repeat.

ROTATE WRIST AND PRESS
- Stand up or sit at the edge of a chair. Your feet should be shoulder width apart, arms by your sides, head straight and looking forward.
- Put your hands in fist position, with the insides of your fists facing inward toward your shoulders, at shoulder height, with your elbows close to your body.
- Rotate your wrists, with your fists facing outward, and press your fists into the air overhead by straightening your arms.
- Slowly rotate your wrists back in and return your fists to your shoulders, in the starting position.
- Repeat.

SEATED ROW
- Sit at the edge of a chair with your feet shoulder width apart and your arms at your sides.
- Slightly hinge over at the waist with your hands in fist position and your arms straight in a diagonal position past your knees.
- Keeping your back flat and your core engaged and tight, pull your elbows back and squeeze your shoulder blades.
- Lower your arms back down into starting position.
- Repeat.

TRICEPS KICKBACKS
- Stand up or sit at the edge of a chair. Your feet should be shoulder width apart, arms by your sides, head straight and looking forward.
- Keeping your back straight, slightly hinge over at the waist with your hands in fist position.

- Keep your head up and your arms bent at your side so that your arms are aligned closely to your body, forming a 90-degree angle. This is your starting position.
- Using only your triceps, exhale as you extend your arms fully backward, bringing them nearly parallel with the floor.
- Repeat.

CIRCUIT 3

ANKLE (SHIN) HINGE OVERS
- Sit at the edge of a chair with your feet shoulder width apart and your arms at your sides.
- Hinge over at the waist, back straight, head neutral, and eyes up, with arms straight and hands reaching toward your ankles or shins, keeping your back flat and your core engaged and tight.
- Then rise up and return to the starting position.
- Repeat.

SINGLE-ARM ROTATIONAL UPWARD PUNCH (RIGHT SIDE)
- Stand up or sit at the edge of a chair. Your feet should be shoulder width apart, arms by your sides, head straight and looking forward. Curl your hands into fists.
- Raise your fists in front of your shoulders.
- Simultaneously step your left leg out to the side a little past shoulder width, rotate your torso, and punch your left arm into the air diagonally toward the right, straightening your arm.
- Then, simultaneously, bring your left leg and left arm back to the starting position.
- Repeat.

SEATED CRUNCH

- Sit at the edge of a chair with your feet shoulder width apart and place your hands behind your ears, your elbows out to the sides and rounded slightly in. Suck in your navel toward your spine and engage your abs. This will be your starting position.
- Crunch your upper body down while fully exhaling. Intentionally squeeze your abs. Allow your upper back to round while avoiding any movement in your lower back. Imagine that you have a string attached from your shoulders to your hips that suddenly shortens. The crunching move is subtle and shouldn't be exaggerated.
- While keeping your abs contracted, return to your sitting position. Inhale on your way up.
- Go directly into the next repetition without releasing your abdominal muscles.
- Repeat.

ANKLE (SHIN) HINGE OVERS TO HAMMER CURL

- Sit at the edge of a chair with your feet shoulder width apart and your arms at your sides, curling your hands into fists.
- Hinge over at the waist, back straight, head neutral, and eyes up, with arms straight and fists facing each other, shoulder width apart, reaching toward your ankles or shins, keeping your back flat and your core engaged and tight.
- Simultaneously rise up, keeping your upper arms stable and shoulders relaxed, and bend at the elbow and bring your fists toward your shoulders. Your elbows should stay tucked in close to your ribs.
- Lower your arms back to your sides.
- Repeat.

ALTERNATING ROTATIONAL UPWARD PUNCHES
(TO THE LEFT SIDE)

- Stand up or sit at the edge of a chair. Your feet should be shoulder width apart, arms by your sides, head straight and looking forward. Curl your hands into fists.
- Raise your fists in front of your shoulders.
- Whether you are sitting or standing, step your right leg out to the side a little past shoulder width, rotate your torso, and punch your right arm into the air diagonally toward the left, straightening your arm.
- Then simultaneously bring your right leg and right arm back to the starting position.
- Repeat, switching sides.

SEATED CRUNCH PULSE

- Sit at the edge of a chair with your feet shoulder width apart and place your hands behind your ears, your elbows out to the sides, rounded slightly in. Suck in your navel toward your spine and engage your abs. This will be your starting position.
- Crunch your upper body down while fully exhaling. Intentionally squeeze your abs. Allow your upper back to round while avoiding any movement in your lower back. Imagine that you have a string attached from your shoulders to your hips that suddenly shortens. Then stay in position and crunch quickly in short pulses.
- Repeat.

ANKLE (SHIN) HINGE OVERS TO HAMMER CURL TO PRESS

- Sit at the edge of a chair with your feet shoulder width apart and your arms at your sides, hands in fist position.

- Hinge over at the waist, back straight, head neutral, and eyes up, with arms straight and fists facing each other, shoulder width apart, reaching toward your ankles or shins, keeping your back flat and your core engaged and tight.
- Simultaneously rise up, keeping your upper arms stable and your shoulders relaxed, and bend at the elbow and bring your fists toward your shoulders. Your elbows should stay tucked in close to your ribs.
- Raise your arms above head and extend your elbows, with your fists facing each other.
- Lower your fists back to your shoulders, unfolding your elbows, with your arms returning to your sides.
- Repeat.

CIRCUIT 4

CLASP OVERHEAD TRICEPS
- Stand up or sit at the edge of a chair. Your feet should be shoulder width apart, arms extended directly overhead with hands clasped.
- Keeping your chest up, core engaged, and back straight, bend your elbows and lower your clasped hands behind your head without moving your upper arms.
- Pause, and then unfold elbows and press your clasped hands back up to the starting position.

SINGLE-SIDE RUSSIAN TWIST (RIGHT)
- Stand up or sit at the edge of a chair. Your feet should be shoulder width apart. Place your hands in front of your chest, link them together, then brace your core and lean back as close to a 45-degree angle as possible.

- Bring your arms all the way toward the right, then return to the center.
- Repeat.

LATERAL RAISE TO FRONT RAISE

- Stand up or sit at the edge of a chair. Your feet should be shoulder width apart and your arms at your sides, curling your hands into fists.
- Check your posture, roll your shoulders back, engage your core, and look straight ahead.
- Raise your arms simultaneously up and out to each side, keeping your arms almost completely straight, stopping when your elbows reach shoulder height and your body is forming a T shape. Breathe in as you lift.
- Pause and hold for a second at the top of the movement.
- Lower your arms slowly, bringing your arms back to your sides. Breathe out as you lower your arms.
- Then raise your arms simultaneously up and in front, keeping your arms almost completely straight at shoulder height. Breathe in as you lift.
- Pause and hold for a second at the top of the movement.
- Lower your arms slowly, bringing your arms back to your sides. Breathe out as you lower your arms.
- Repeat.

SINGLE-SIDE RUSSIAN TWIST (LEFT)

- Stand up or sit at the edge of a chair. Your feet should be shoulder width apart. Place your hands in front of your chest, link them together, then brace your core and lean back as close to a 45-degree angle as possible.

- Bring your arms all the way toward the left, then return to the center.
- Repeat.

LATERAL RAISE TO FRONT RAISE TO BACK SQUEEZE
- Stand up or sit at the edge of a chair. Your feet should be shoulder width apart and your arms at your sides, curling your hands into fists.
- Check your posture, roll your shoulders back, engage your core, and look straight ahead.
- Raise your arms simultaneously up and out to each side, keeping your arms almost completely straight, stopping when your elbows reach shoulder height and your body is forming a T shape. Breathe in as you lift.
- Pause and hold for a second at the top of the movement.
- Lower your arms slowly, bringing your arms back to your sides. Breathe out as you lower your arms.
- Then raise your arms simultaneously up and in front, keeping your arms almost completely straight at shoulder height. Breathe in as you lift.
- Pause and hold for a second at the top of the movement.
- Then bend your elbows back, squeezing your shoulder blades. Hold for a second.
- Then return your arms out to the front and lower your arms slowly, bringing your arms back to your sides. Breathe out as you lower your arms.
- Repeat.

DOUBLE-SIDE RUSSIAN TWIST (RIGHT TO LEFT)
- Stand up or sit at the edge of a chair. Your feet should be shoulder width apart. Place your hands in front of your chest, link

them together, then brace your core and lean back as close to a 45-degree angle as possible.

- Bring your arms all the way toward the right, then return to the center, then bring your arms all the way toward the left, and finally, return to center.
- That is one rep. Repeat.

ACTIVITIES OUTSIDE THE HOME

Outings can be either beneficial or disruptive. If your LO is really committed to their schedule, breaking it up with an outing may increase their agitation. Or they may love to break up the monotony of staying indoors or being at home. The general rule is to meet your LO where they are: start by planning an entire day outside the home with a destination, like a museum or the beach, and see how they respond. Then, as they decline, adjust the duration and event: instead of a whole day at a museum, take it down to dinner at a restaurant.

Use the same approach to timing as well. Go out when your LO is at their peak energy and attention. Outings should always be supervised, as even in the earliest stages, your LO could get lost in a familiar place, or panic that they won't be able to get home. They must always wear their ID bracelet, too, in case you become separated.

Outings include doctor appointments; personal grooming (the hairdresser, barber, or nail salon); going to their church or house of worship; visiting family and friends; or entertainment, like a park, a museum, a dance performance, a movie, or a ball game. Wherever you choose, plan for extra time to get there and have an exit strategy if your LO becomes overwhelmed or overtired. Most importantly, take advantage of opportunities as they come up, because in the late stages of the disease, leaving home will become too agitating. I had always wanted to take my aunt to see a play on Broadway, but by the time I was able to take her, her disease had progressed and she wasn't able to sit in a theater for 2-plus hours.

Incorporating the Arts into the Family Care Plan

People with dementia/AD can continue to connect with the arts regardless of what stage they're in, which will provide a multitude of sensory experiences. In the early stages, attend a live performance or gallery outing, and later, bring the experience home with books and video programming. Museums all over the world offer virtual tours, or you can sign up for virtual art or music appreciation classes. These are activities you and your LO can do together and then talk about.

TRAVELING IN THE REAL WORLD

In the earliest stages, your LO may still be working and/or driving. Deciding when to end those activities is a personal decision, yet you should start to take safety into account immediately. Older drivers in general are at higher risk for getting into an accident and getting lost, and these risks are only compounded with dementia/AD. At the very least, you and your LO should be linked through a GPS app on your phone so that you know where they are at all times. There will come a time when it becomes clear that your LO should no longer be driving: it will probably be obvious, as the car may have new dents, or your LO may tell you that they've recently been ticketed for driving too slowly. At that point, you are going to have to deliver the news, and enforce the policy, that driving is now off the table.

I do not recommend that anyone with dementia/AD—regardless of what stage they are in—travel alone, either to work or for leisure. What's more, they should not be taking public transportation or a rideshare, either. If your LO is in the earlier stages and they are working outside the home, work into the Family Care Plan time to drive them to work, or have them driven by someone on your team. If you need to take your LO somewhere and you don't have a ride, be proactive and look into transportation services their community provides ahead of time. Some of these options may take months to put in place because of demand and the need for preapproval. Anyone who is accompanying your LO to an appointment or activity is entitled to receive this service.

If long-distance travel is necessary, pick the shortest route and most efficient transportation options whenever possible. For people with dementia/AD, traveling can be excessively stimulating, especially if they are going to or through a noisy place, like an airport or train station. Airports are a perfect storm for a dementia meltdown: they are chaotic, crowded, and loud. One way to make the trip less stressful is by limiting distractions. Narrow your LO's field of vision with sunglasses that block peripheral vision, and offer them earplugs.

If you have to fly, consider enrolling yourself and your LO in TSA PreCheck, which will put you on a shorter security line. The Transportation Security Administration (TSA) also offers additional assistance through their program TSA Cares (855-787-2227). Call three days ahead of a scheduled flight and tell them you are traveling with someone who has dementia/AD. A representative will meet you on the entry side of security and help you through the process. When you and your LO go through security, you should go through the metal detector first. This will ensure that you and your LO aren't separated.

Individual airlines offer services like wheelchairs to the boarding area, early boarding, and more. You can arrange for these services when you purchase your tickets online through the airline's own website. Make sure these arrangements carry through to every leg of your trip. If you are traveling to visit friends or family, remember to take your LO's needs into account. Seeing new faces will be both exciting and anxiety-producing. What's more, your LO will be off their regular routine. While staying with friends and family may seem like a way to get others to pitch in with the caregiving or save money, you will be putting a burden on your host that they may not be prepared for, and making life more complicated for your LO. Instead, I recommend that you book a hotel room close by so you and your LO can retreat to your own space when you need to wind down. When you get to your destination, greet everyone, and then make a quick exit to the hotel and set up the room so that you can attempt to re-create your Family Care Plan.

SOCIALIZATION OPPORTUNITIES

The last part of your Family Care Plan activity roundup is socialization. Just like Mel, your LO needs to engage with people (besides you), and often. That's another reason why the team approach is key: when you schedule in your LO's friends and family, you are automatically making sure that they stay socially engaged in the safest way possible.

Outside the home, use adult daycare and other programs for people with dementia/AD. For example, in New York City a group called the Unforgettables is a chorus made up of people with dementia and

Doctor Appointments Are Activities

Every time you leave the home with your LO, you are doing an activity. This includes doctor visits. As I've said, whenever possible, schedule all your doctor appointments on the same day of the week so that you can maintain control over your care plan.

Even in the early stages, you must accompany your LO to the doctor. Once, I was in a doctor's office waiting room, and I noticed an elderly couple struggling for 20 minutes with the intake forms. From the way they were talking to each other it was clear to me that they both had early-stage dementia. The whole scenario was upsetting; this couple should never have come to see their physician without someone to assist them. If they couldn't fill out the forms, how were they going to understand their doctor's instructions?

Your LO may not want to see their doctor as often as is truly needed. I always choose the carrot over the stick. Plan for a fun treat afterward, whether it's ice cream, a meal out, or window-shopping. And don't be surprised if both of you are tired after the appointment; it can be hard work just trying to make sense of what a doctor is saying.

their caregivers. There may be a similar offering near you, and if not, ask your church's or town's social services agency to consider putting one together.

Your LO's house of worship may also offer socialization opportunities. Religious services, pastoral visits, or clubs can be uplifting ways to spend the day—or a few hours—outside the home, and let's not forget about spiritual music! There may also be a group made up of church members that provide friendly visits, which can continue through all of the stages of the disease. If your LO was involved in a house of worship or any other community service, make sure that they can keep up with those activities until they can't any longer.

Activities Take Time

As you modify your Family Care Plan and schedule activities, leave plenty of room for setting them up and closing them down, or for leaving the home. Everything you do with your LO may seem like it is in slow motion, but remember that they are going as fast as they can.

CHAPTER 7

Dealing with Difficult Behaviors

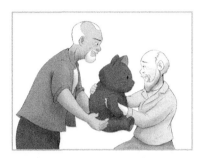

I once worked for Irma, a woman whose daughter kept telling me that her mother had been a high-achieving educator and was recently diagnosed with early-stage dementia. Irma's daughter, Tanya, told me that her mother had always been well-mannered, and now she was "completely crazy" and particularly combative with relatives who came into the house. Tanya was at her wits' end and couldn't manage her mother and her full-time job. That was when she brought me into the home.

Once I assessed Irma, I knew right away that the problem wasn't as simple as a late-in-life personality switch. Instead, I could see that her mother was frustrated. The daughter was still in denial and had not recognized the significant amount of help Irma needed with her day-to-day life, even in the early stages of the disease, and had taken to flitting in and out of the house after a cursory check-in around breakfast time. Once Irma understood that she would have the help she needed from me, I was able to manage the rest of the family members, giving them specific tasks that would make her life run more smoothly. Within a week, her bad behavior toward them subsided.

Many of the new caregivers I talk to worry about the "acting-out behaviors" that are all too common for people with dementia/AD. The truth is, the way that the caregiver approaches a difficult situation often escalates their reactions. What's more, bad behaviors do not come out of nowhere; there's usually an underlying cause that can be addressed to make the behavior go away.

No one is expecting you to be on your best behavior with your LO all the time. However, if you see that your LO is resorting to the same antagonistic responses, there is probably a better way to deal with them. The goal is to curb your LO's agitation and disruptiveness so that they can return to behaving like themselves, which will make you feel less distressed. The tools that I provide in this chapter will lessen your stress levels because they will prepare you for what's to come—and how to respond.

The first step to is to identify exactly what's happening by keeping notes in your Daily Observation, and what has worked, and not worked, in the past to mitigate them. Use the same assessment strategy from Chapter 5:

- *Describe:* Write down exactly what are you seeing, as in *"Mom threw her pillows at me when I told her to get out of bed,"* or *"Dad yelled at me to 'stop bothering him' when I reminded him to use the bathroom."*

- *Measure:* There are actual, scientific scales that rate the behaviors in people with dementia/AD to determine if they require medication to control problematic incidences. These are called the Behavioral Pathology in Alzheimer's Disease Rating Scale (BEHAVE-AD), the BEHAVE-AD Frequency-Weighted Severity Scale (BEHAVE-AD-FW), and the Empirical BEHAVE-AD Rating Scale (E-BEHAVE-AD). Your LO's doctor may discuss these scales with you, so your notes that measure how one outburst compares to another are critically important. You can use a rating scale that ranges from one to ten whenever you are performing an observation, where one is a mild, nonphysical reaction and ten is a total behavioral meltdown, including a physical component such as biting, scratching, spitting, hitting, and so on.

- *Conditions:* Record the conditions under which the behavior occurred. When this behavior occurs, what else is happening? Was the mother in the example above sound asleep? Were the father's pants already wet?

- *Time frame:* How long did the behavior last?

- *Details:* Include as many details as possible! This will help you see trends in what has worked, and what hasn't, in terms of fixing the behavior.

Then make a plan. It's very hard to change tactics *in the moment.* Write down how you think you should handle the situation next time based on the following suggestions. Lastly, evaluate: When you were able to put your plan into action, did it work? It can take a few days to see if your intervention altered the response even temporarily. If the strategy worked, share it with the rest of your team. If not, try a new approach next time.

NAME THAT BEHAVIOR

Changes in your LO's personality can be exasperating, frightening, and sometimes physically painful, but they do not come out of nowhere. Dementia/AD destroys brain cells, which means that the connections between those cells are no longer robust. Not only does this loss result in forgetfulness, it results in the loss of behavioral memory; your LO simply does not remember how to appropriately behave. This is the reason why they may exhibit behaviors that are not typical of their previous personality. I can't tell you how many times I have been caring for someone and their children will tell me, *"I'm so embarrassed; Mom never acted like this before."* The good news is that by curbing these issues, your LO may be able to act, and feel, more like themselves.

AVOIDANCE AND RESISTING

Avoidance is any refusal to do something, like eat, get out of bed, or get dressed. It can also look like self-isolating; sometimes people won't leave their room even when you are living with them, or they can speak but they won't speak to you. These uncooperative behaviors can be caused by physical or emotional discomfort. For instance, if your LO's dentures are making eating painful, they may not be able to convey this and just refuse to eat. Or perhaps this behavior occurs when there isn't an established daily routine, or if the routine was disturbed. First, make sure that your LO isn't in physical pain, and if they are, address it immediately (see Chapter 8). Then revisit your Family Care Plan and get back on track. Using the calm communication style that you mastered in Chapter 5, give short instructions rather than asking questions or for permission.

If your LO is refusing to get up, showered, and dressed, focus on the most necessary aspect of the routine and accomplish that first, skipping the rest for later. In this instance, if you need to get your LO ready for an appointment, they can always shower later in the day. If they refuse, try again in a few minutes.

Reinforce completing the task with a prize: *"Thanks for getting dressed. Let's have your favorite breakfast,"* or *"Take your medicine and later we'll go for ice cream."*

COMBATIVENESS—VERBAL ASSAULTS

Your LO may say something mean, make a hurtful accusation, or just start screaming. These verbal assaults often occur when they are frustrated or in distress and unable to express what's bothering them. In most cases, your LO isn't really upset at you, so try to not take what they are saying personally. In every way, this is the same acting-out behavior that you see in toddlers when they can't use their words to explain what's going on.

First, make sure that your LO isn't in physical pain, and if they are, address it immediately (see Chapter 8). Then lower the volume of your environment—literally. Turn off any extraneous noises or stimuli, like the television. A soft touch on their arm or shoulder combined with an even-toned voice can help calm them down. Make eye contact with a pleasant facial expression. All of these are signals that you are in control.

Next, redirect by focusing on an activity you know they love, as in *"Mom, you don't need to yell at me, I'm right here. Let's look at the family photos."* Or prompt them to tell you about their deep past, like their childhood. For example, *"Marcus, I love this black-and-white photograph on the dresser. Tell me about it."* Either of these redirection prompts opens up an opportunity for your LO to use their memory and feel good about it. When they are calmer, they may be able to tell you what's really bothering them. If the combativeness continues, assume that you haven't resolved the situation. No matter what, do not scream back.

Another strategy to defuse the situation is to avoid engaging altogether (after you make sure that they are not in physical distress). Sometimes any communication can agitate a person with dementia/AD. Instead, let them rant. After a few minutes, your LO should be able to calm themselves down, at which point you can offer a short directive to move them in another direction. For example, if your LO is agitated after lunch, use a short directive, combined with physical touch. Try *"Let's take a shower."*

A change of scenery—even if it's just another room in the home—can improve their mood, too, as can regular physical activity, like walking or even gardening and soft music. Just like you use music to de-stress, you will find it an excellent way to manage your LO's agitation, irritability, and aggression during any stage of dementia/AD. My client Joanne would become combative about once a day, seemingly for no reason. The first thing I would do was walk away from her and put on her favorite music. When she heard the music, it brought her back to a better time, and she was able to soothe herself.

Some people with dementia/AD may self-soothe by sucking on candy, chewing gum, or even smoking cigarettes. Of course, smoking is the most dangerous of these habits for a number of reasons. Your LO should smoke only when you are right there in the room with them.

COMBATIVENESS—PHYSICAL ASSAULTS

People with dementia/AD resort to a range of negative physical behaviors, including grabbing, kicking, pushing, hitting, throwing things, and biting. You may be surprised how strong your LO is, and how much pain they can inflict. I once worked with a client named Pearl who would hit and lash out when she was sitting at the dining table right before lunch or dinner. (Oddly, she was well-behaved for breakfast.) She would take her fork and jab family members as they passed her. Physical assaults often stem from the same issues as verbal combativeness: something is bothering or frustrating your LO. Stay calm and back away; do not engage or hit back. If you are stronger than they are, take a deep breath and talk them down in a gentle manner. Try not to take the behavior personally. Use open body language: keep your arms at your sides instead of crossed over your body, and do not raise your hands, which they may misinterpret as a threat.

Then try to identify the immediate cause or trigger of the behavior and focus on addressing your LO's feelings and the situation rather than the hitting. Determine if they are in pain. In Pearl's case, I observed that her dentures weren't sitting in her mouth correctly. Breakfast was always a softer meal, so that didn't bother her, but lunch and dinner were tougher on her gums and teeth, and chewing was painful. She was acting out her discomfort during these meals and trying to get our attention by using her fork as a weapon.

When the episode is over, take care of yourself. See if you are bleeding or bruised and treat your wounds. Then assess the environment and determine where you can make changes. We replaced Pearl's sharp silverware with plastic and cut her food into tiny pieces in the kitchen before we brought it to the table (you'll learn more about this strategy in Chapter 9). This was enough of a fix until we could get her to the dentist and have her dentures reset. Other tools I've used to limit physicality include chewing gum, stress balls, music, playing with Velcro darts, and wrapping the person in a weighted blanket.

If you are smaller than your LO and feel like you are in danger, call 911. Even if they have not assaulted you yet, contact your local police to let them know that your LO has been diagnosed with dementia/AD and may be a problem in the future. Alerting the police in advance that your LO has dementia/AD may influence how they respond if they are ever called to the home.

If your LO has a history of violence, they will require 24-hour supervision even in the earliest stages—for their own safety as well as the safety of anyone who comes in contact with them.

Is Your LO Signaling an Unmet Need?

Disruptive or odd behaviors may be a sign that your LO has a need that is not being addressed. When they are presenting with any type of challenging behaviors, consider if your LO could be:

- Hungry or thirsty
- In an environment that is too bright, too dark, or too noisy
- In pain
- Irritated by their clothing
- Requiring a trip to the bathroom, or just had an accident
- Tired
- Too hot or too cold
- Emotionally distressed: angry, sad, lonely, scared, or bored

---

DEPRESSION/APATHY

Ava became depressed after she socialized with family and friends. She was able to express that she was sad because she couldn't keep up with the conversations. This is not unusual; your LO may understand their limitations and feel crummy about it. They may also express apathy if they are bored. If they are severely depressed and talking about death or suicide, do not take these cues lightly. Have your LO seen by their doctor, who may prescribe antidepressants and/or therapy.

In the moment, you can try to break a depressive or apathetic cycle by redirecting your LO to a physical activity, such as going outside for a walk. Fresh air and exercise are a potent combination for improving mood. On the walk, talk with your LO about how they are feeling, which will show them not only that you care but that you are taking their feelings and thoughts into consideration. Knowing that they have been heard can also help them feel more in control.

Afterward, make sure that your LO is sleeping well, that they are fully hydrated, and that their meals are nutritious and have plenty of vitamin B (see Chapter 9). Check their medications to see if depression is a side effect or a sign of an improper dosage. Work more physical and mental stimulation into the Family Care Plan, and increase socializing opportunities that are appropriate for their stage.

FORGETFULNESS

Remington is my friend's husband, in his seventies. After he retired, he started going for a daily neighborhood walk in the afternoon. About two months into this new routine, Remington noticed he was getting confused and lost during his walk. He would wait until he ran into someone to ask for directions back home.

Forgetfulness is a typical early-stage behavior that can lead to agitation and frustration. When it happens, sit your LO down and give them the time and space to remember what it is they forgot: it's likely they will eventually remember. Don't correct them, and don't ask questions as prompts. Instead, offer to find whatever is lost or forgotten, together. Then set up procedures so that things don't go by the wayside in the future, such as creating a specific place for house keys.

Medications That May Cause Depression

The following drugs may cause depression, especially in the elderly:[1]

- Anticonvulsants: Drugs used to control epileptic seizures. These include ethosuximide (Zarontin) and methsuximide (Celontin).
- Barbiturates: Depressants that slow brain function and are used to treat anxiety and to prevent epileptic seizures. These include phenobarbital and secobarbital.
- Benzodiazepines: Another group of depressants used to treat anxiety and insomnia and as a muscle relaxant. These include alprazolam (Xanax), clonazepam (Klonopin), chlordiazepoxide (Librium), diazepam (Valium), flurazepam (Dalmane), lorazepam (Ativan), and triazolam (Halcion).
- Beta-adrenergic blockers: Drugs used for treating migraine headaches and heart problems, including high blood pressure, heart failure, chest pain, and abnormal heart rhythms. These include atenolol (Tenormin), carvedilol (Coreg), and metoprolol (Lopressor).
- Calcium-channel blockers: Another class of heart medication that treat high blood pressure, chest pain, congestive heart failure, and abnormal heart rhythms. These include diltiazem (Cardizem, Tiazac), nifedipine (Procardia), and verapamil (Calan).
- Interferon alfa: A drug used to treat certain cancers and hepatitis B and C.
- Opioids: Drugs used to relieve pain. These include codeine, meperidine (Demerol), morphine, and oxycodone (OxyContin).
- Statins: Drugs used to lower cholesterol and prevent heart attacks. These include atorvastatin (Lipitor), fluvastatin (Lescol), pravastatin (Pravachol), and simvastatin (Zocor).

I suggested that Remington get a classy ID bracelet that he would feel good about wearing. About a week later it came in handy, because someone noticed that he was confused and called his wife. Afterward, she made sure to go on his daily walk with him.

HALLUCINATIONS

Hallucinations are associated with Lewy body dementia, although people with other dementia diagnoses can also experience them. My aunt used to tell me that there were children in her bedroom, and of course, there weren't.

In many instances, hallucinations aren't disturbing for the people experiencing them (although they can lead to acting out during dreaming, and even sleepwalking, which can be dangerous). If this is the case, I don't think that there is much to gain by correcting your LO. However, if the hallucinations are scary, they are worthy of investigation. If there are shadows that could be misinterpreted, eliminate them by moving furniture or changing the lighting. If there is no clear basis for the hallucinations, have your LO evaluated by a neurologist, who may prescribe antipsychotic medications like risperidone, or even cannabis products that contain cannabidiol (CBD).

HOARDING

People with dementia/AD love to collect stuff they believe they may need some day. I find the behavior kind of sweet until it takes over a room or becomes smelly or dirty. My client Sophia stockpiled empty water bottles and did not want anyone to dispose of them. When I asked her why, she told me that she wanted to take them to the supermarket to collect the deposit money. That seemed reasonable, but then I discovered that she was also collecting bottle caps and stashing them in cups and flowerpots and in the corners of her room.

If hoarding behaviors give your LO a sense of control, just go with it. Let them use their special closet (see Chapter 4) to keep their collection in one place. You can also make an activity of sorting their items or creating scrapbooks.

However, if it is negatively impacting your home by taking up too much space or attracting bugs or rodents, throw the stuff away when they are distracted with another activity. Don't go halfway and only throw out some, because they will notice. If they ask where their collection is, use a beneficial fib: *"I've sent it out to be cleaned."*

OVERSEXUALIZED BEHAVIORS

These behaviors can occur in both men and women with dementia/AD and are linked to boredom, discomfort, anxiety, or distress. I've seen people in memory care centers take off all their clothes in public only to find out that they were simply too hot and not really looking for lovin'.

If you are a caregiver for your spouse, be patient with them when they are feeling amorous, even if you aren't. Give extra reassurances that you love them and the physical contact they may need by snuggling in the morning or before going to sleep, being available and present for hugs, kisses, a massage, and even dancing together.

However, some sexual advances are disturbing. One man that I cared for named Winston no longer recognized his wife and would approach her suggestively as a stranger. We decided that the best course of action was to alter sleeping arrangements, with the two of them in separate rooms.

If your LO is bothering you for sexual favors (and you are not their spouse or partner), stay calm and be patient. With kindness, tell your LO that you are not interested. Don't send mixed signals, like allowing the behavior one time and then reacting negatively the next time. Consider dressing your LO in adaptive clothing jumpsuits that snap in the back, which will be harder for them to remove. If you catch your LO masturbating, gently ask them to find a more private setting, like their bedroom or the bathroom. Keep notes on inappropriate sexual behaviors so that you can determine the triggers. For instance, you may notice that Mom or Dad touches themselves when they need to use the bathroom.

Then distract them and redirect them to another, positive activity.

Why Robotic Therapy Pets Work

Eldercare researchers have found that pets, alive or robotic, help to retrieve old emotions and memories for people with dementia/ AD. When the emotions are positive, they can momentarily help your LO focus, decreasing stress and anxiety and pushing aside the sense of disorientation that they are continuously struggling with. They are so effective that studies have shown that the person may require less medication for anxiety and pain.[2]

Robotic pets provide all the upside of a real pet without the extra burden of their care. They've been around since 2003 and are approved by the Food and Drug Administration (FDA). They imitate specific animal behaviors with movements and vocalizations, and they respond to light, sound, temperature, and touch. The newest models have artificial intelligence features that allow these robots to develop their own personalities and respond to your LO in unique ways.

In this case, give your LO something to do with their hands, like working with clay or holding a fidget toy or stuffed animal. If they like babies and/or pets, consider getting a robotic therapy doll. However, not everyone likes babies or pets, even when they are pretend, so watch how your LO reacts and adjust accordingly.

PARANOIA OR DELUSIONAL BEHAVIORS

Paranoia is intricately linked to dementia/AD. Your LO may forget where they put something and assume that it was stolen. Or they hide their belongings to protect them. I've worked with many women with AD who sleep with their purses tucked into their beds.

I've found that there's little to gain in correcting your LO, because no matter how hard you try, you will never be able to prove that you haven't taken the item they are protecting (or misplaced!). Instead, find a place for them—like a special closet—to store the things they are paranoid about losing. Then redirect them to another activity or conversation.

Sometimes your LO's paranoia is based in reality. They may be looking for something that you have stored away, even if they were part of the conversation when you packed it up. It's a good idea to make a list of what's no longer in the home. Then, when they are in a calm state, show your LO the list and reassure them that these items are safe.

REGRESSIVE LIVING (FOCUSING ON THE PAST)

Steven's grandmother had dementia and at age 98 was spending the last few years of her life reliving the high school musicals that she had been in. At first these conversations were alarming to her family, but the truth is, this is expected behavior. People with dementia/AD can recall the distant past with clarity compared to yesterday or last week or last year. By being a good listener, you may learn something wonderful and new about your LO instead of becoming frustrated that they aren't living in the moment.

Most of their regressions return them to pleasant memories. However, if you find that your LO is being haunted by something traumatic, they will need more than a good listener. Take notes and present the information to their primary care physician and/or neurologist and see if they recommend a therapist.

REPETITIVE QUESTIONING

Every caregiver has a story about how their LO asked them the same question a thousand times over the course of a day, an afternoon, or even an hour. Unfortunately, repetitive questioning, which is considered an anxious behavior, comes with the territory. Sharing your calendar or care plan and the activities to expect over the next few days can help cut down on it. Remove visual cues that may make your LO anxious. Put away keys, purses, and coats until they are needed. Fidget toys and blankets can be calming, as can a change of scenery or an engaging activity like an art project.

SPEECH AND COMMUNICATION DIFFICULTIES

Speech and communication problems seem to set in most severely outside the home, because when you're at home and have each other's complete attention, you can probably communicate even when they can't find their words. Once, my client Wyatt was at a doctor appointment and wasn't able to express that he was no longer sleeping well. When the doctor started asking questions, Wyatt just stared into the distance. I could tell from his expression that he could not conceptualize what the doctor was saying or communicate his confusion.

If speech problems occur outside the home, end the outing and return to a more familiar environment. This will alleviate any frustration that is building. If they occur suddenly in the home, it may be that your LO is overtired, uncomfortable, dehydrated, or sliding into the next stage of the disease. One recent study counterintuitively suggested that individuals with AD, even in the latest stages, communicate more clearly and better understand what is being said to them when lively music with a fast tempo is playing in the background.[3] It's worth a try as long as the music isn't so loud that your LO or you have to scream over it to be heard.

SUNDOWNING

Sundowning is a signature symptom of dementia/AD characterized by confusion, anxiety, agitation, ignoring directions, restlessness, pacing, wandering, and yelling in the late afternoon and early evening. It occurs most frequently in the moderate and late stages. It is one of the most distressing behaviors for caregivers to deal with because it can happen with such regularity, no matter how many times you try to correct it.

There are four ways to address sundowning behaviors. First, make sure your LO is well rested and adhering to a sleep schedule (see Chapter 8) that includes few opportunities for daytime naps. Increase the light in your home during the day, and keep your home darker at night. Give them the space they need to have their meltdown as safely as possible. Lastly, reassure them that this feeling of despondency will pass, and distract them with a favorite activity. Calming music, especially from your LO's past, is helpful in reversing this behavior in the moment.

I'm also a huge fan of allowing my patients to interact with animals, which has been shown to decrease anxiety, confusion, and agitation. Many organizations will come to your home with a therapy animal and a trained handler, and you can schedule it for the time your LO is usually the most anxious. This activity provides emotional, social, and cognitive benefits for any stage of the disease.

WANDERING

Wandering and sundowning seem to go hand-in-hand. I've found that covering doorknobs with a cloth that is the same color as the door can prevent your LO from getting very far, because they will not be able to see the doorknob. Remove triggers for leaving as discussed earlier, like keeping keys and coats away from the door. Some people go as far as disguising their front door with a poster or a piece of artwork. I've also found that putting on familiar music seems to be soothing when people with dementia/AD are feeling restless or start to wander.

If your LO looks like they are ready to leave home or walk away from you, ask them where they are going, who they are looking for, and what they need. They may be able to tell you what's troubling them. In this case, remind them where they are and that they are safe. Make sure they are getting enough exercise, so that they use unspent energy and are able to release their stress earlier in the day. A rummage box can hold their attention, or sitting them in a chair that has a unique textured fabric.

Some memory centers set up a "bus stop to nowhere" outside their building. When their clients get agitated, they bring them to the bus stop and tell them that they are going on a trip. Once the patient and caregiver sit at the bus stop for a few minutes, the impulse to wander decreases. You can do the same by accompanying your LO outside when they are ready to wander. It's a counterintuitive strategy that really works.

EMPATHY GOES A LONG WAY

Dealing with these difficult behaviors is by far the hardest part of being a caregiver for someone with dementia/AD. Compared to taking care of someone frail or elderly, your LO is likely to be in otherwise good health. For many caregivers, this can lead to a feeling of *"Why am I still here if my LO is treating me so poorly?"*

On these days, try to remember that your LO needs you, and if they could control their bad behaviors, they would. At the same time, listen for clues. As you've learned, poor behavior is often a signal that something else is going wrong. And if one fix doesn't work, don't hesitate to try another, even on the same day.

Whenever you have extremely stressful days, make sure that you save some time to do something that's just for you. Review the self-care options in Chapter 3 and schedule someone from your team to lend a hand every day.

CHAPTER 8

Identifying and Treating
Common Medical Problems

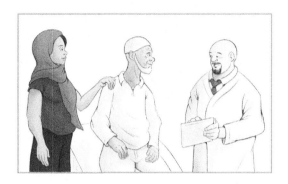

Denial can creep into caregiving when it comes to your LO's physical health, as you may not want to add resolving their other symptoms or conditions to your list of responsibilities. However, as you do your Daily Observation, you'll inevitably notice that your LO is changing. The goal is to address these physical changes as they come up, which is the easiest time to deal with them, before they get worse or cause further health problems.

In this chapter I will show you how to act exactly like a professional nurse when you see that something has gone wrong, whether it's pain, discomfort, or physical decline. The truth is, you don't have to address your LO's mental decline, because it is expected. However, they may have physical complaints that result from dementia/AD behaviors or further impair their cognitive status. By addressing these complaints, you will ensure that your LO is comfortable, less anxious, and able to be in the world to the best of their capability.

The following categories are the most likely places you'll notice physical decline in your LO. If they also have chronic conditions like diabetes or heart disease, their doctor will tell you additional signs and symptoms to look for. We'll discuss what you can do to treat some of these conditions at home, and which symptoms require prompt treatment.

The Internet Is Not an Ideal Medical Resource

The Internet is chock-full of information, and it's tempting to use it as a first-line resource when your LO is struggling or in pain. However, *it's not the only resource available to you.* Medical information on the Internet is not always up-to-date, and you may also find conflicting information or descriptions of individual experiences that have nothing to do with your LO, or worse, advice that is not medically sound or just plain inappropriate.

Instead, use this book as a starting point for care. Then, when you have more questions—and you will—take the time to speak to a medical professional.

APPETITE CHANGES/WEIGHT LOSS

Many people with dementia lose weight. In the earliest stages, your LO may simply forget to eat a meal, or skip one if they can't figure out how to prepare it. In the moderate stages, your LO may burn off more calories during the day because of frequent pacing and fidgeting. Other issues with their health, like hearing, vision, or dental problems, can make eating less pleasurable. In the later stages, they may lose their ability to swallow and chew as their muscles and reflexes no longer work properly.

While you may not think that weight loss is a serious problem, for someone with dementia/AD, it can be. Being underweight affects the immune system and makes it harder for your LO to fight infections. It can also affect their energy levels and their muscle strength, which increases their risk of harm during a fall. If you are weighing your LO weekly and notice that they have lost an average of two pounds a week in recent months, you need to address the situation.

If your LO starts to lose weight, it can be very stressful for the caregiver. Yet turning to tactics like force feeding, constant nudging, and, at end of life, tube feeding, may have no impact. Unfortunately, excessive weight loss is another aspect of this illness and not a failure on your part. However, there are several ways to guide your LO to the table and make eating less difficult and unpleasant.

First, determine why they are losing weight. Depression, pain, fatigue, and lack of physical activity all lead to a poor appetite. Sensory overstimulation—foods that smell too strong or are too spicy or coarse—as well as some medications can affect appetite as well. If they are not interested in the food you are presenting, see if they prefer something else, including a softer option. Introduce a supplemental protein drink between meals, and increase snacks like healthy smoothies, flavored yogurt, or soft fruits. In the next chapter we focus on healthy eating, but if your LO is losing weight, don't worry about giving them more of the foods they love, like ice cream or milkshakes, unless they have underlying food-related health concerns, like diabetes. Your LO's total health always needs to be taken into consideration.

If your LO is having difficulty chewing or swallowing, they need to be seen by a doctor, who may recommend a speech/language therapist or a nutritionist/dietitian. In the meantime, offer food throughout the day and make sure that they keep drinking plenty of water. Chapter 9 focuses on nutrition and mealtime and offers lots of suggestions for getting your LO to eat.

Reevaluate Medications after Weight Loss

If your LO is losing weight between doctor visits, let their doctor know right away. The doctor may order lab work to see if your LO's medication dosages are still correct based on their current weight. You may find that your LO can be taken off certain prescription drugs (such as diabetes- or cholesterol-regulating meds) if they have lost significant weight or their diet has changed.

DEHYDRATION

Your LO may become dehydrated if they're unable to communicate, cannot recognize thirst, or simply forget to drink water. Dehydration leads to headaches, increased confusion and irritability, urinary tract infections, constipation, and fatigue. Typical signs and symptoms of dehydration include dry mouth, sunken eyes, decreased urination, urine that's a darker color than normal, muscle cramping, and dizziness. If your LO's skin loses *turgor*, which is its elasticity, they may be dehydrated. To check, lightly pinch their forearm or abdomen for 1 to 2 seconds: their skin should readily bounce back.

Encourage your LO to drink water throughout the day, shooting for a goal of eight to ten glasses per day. You should be following the same guidelines, so whenever your LO needs to drink a glass, take one as well. Switch up your offerings with hot or iced tea, coffee, fruit juices or smoothies, and soups. Popsicles and flavored ice can help as well; you can purchase sugar-free versions if your LO is diabetic. I love to give my patients the small, 8-ounce water bottles. I find that they will drink them quickly compared to when I give them a 16-ounce size, which they may linger over or never finish.

If your LO is unconscious or severely dehydrated, call 911 immediately. At the hospital, they will receive IV fluid treatments until they are stable enough to return home.

DENTAL PROBLEMS

People in the early stages of dementia/AD often have high levels of plaque, tooth decay, and bleeding or inflamed gums because they have stopped or forgotten their daily dental care routine. They may also have reduced salivary flow due to increased age or dehydration, which causes other dental complications like oral sores and lesions. These issues can also set in during the moderate and later stages, even after you have taken control of their daily care. Dental problems are a particular cause of concern because they can lead to many of the eating problems discussed earlier.

Signs of dental problems include the following:

• Bad breath
• Bleeding or swollen gums after eating, brushing, or flossing
• Clicking/popping noises from the jaw
• Cracked or broken teeth
• Dry mouth
• Ear pain
• Hoarseness
• Jaw swelling
• Loose teeth

- Numbness in the tongue or throat
- Receding gums
- Sensitivity to hot and cold beverages
- Swelling of the face and cheek
- Toothache or pain
- Trouble moving the jaw or tongue
- Trouble swallowing
- Ulcers, sores, or tender areas in the mouth

By following the teeth-brushing directions in Chapter 5, you can put your LO on a better oral care path. They should also see a dentist every six months to check their teeth and, if they wear dentures, to make sure that they are fitting properly.

DIGESTIVE ISSUES

Digestive issues range from constipation to diarrhea and include excessive gas, bloating, and stomach pains. Any of these can cause your LO to feel distressed and uncomfortable, leading to increased anxiety and acting out. If you notice that they are acting differently or holding their stomach, first figure out how their diet may be affecting their health. Are they having enough high-fiber foods, or possibly too much fiber? Are they dehydrated? Are they getting enough exercise over the course of the day?

The first line of treatment is always increasing fluids and finding and eliminating offending foods. In the next chapter, you will learn the ideal diet for your LO, which will be gentler on their digestive system. You can also try over-the-counter medications, but if symptoms persist for a few days, check in with their doctor. Digestive issues may be a sign of more serious illness, including a heart attack or a blood clot in the stomach, called an *embolism*. Digestive issues may also be caused by medications, which can often be switched for another with fewer side effects.

FOOT CARE

A regularly scheduled, professional pedicure not only provides your LO with excellent foot care, it's also an enjoyable outing. The most common foot problems in older adults include gout, bursitis, bunions, hammertoes, and diabetes-related conditions like ulcers. These will be abundantly clear, and will likely have existed well before you became the caregiver. If your LO has any of these conditions, they need to be seen by a podiatrist to manage their care.

Calluses, corns, ingrown nails, thickened or discolored nails, and heel pain can occur at any point, and are caused by general aging, poorly fitting shoes, dry skin, and poor circulation. The skin on the feet can also look cracked, red, swollen, blistered, or peeling, or it can develop a fungus like athlete's foot. Most of these conditions can be resolved with over-the-counter treatments, but if they persist for longer than a week, have your LO see their doctor or a podiatrist.

Swollen feet and ankles may be a sign that your LO is retaining water and needs a diuretic. Or their feet may need to be elevated during the day and in bed, and they need to walk more. Positioning your LO to sleep on their left side helps eliminate fluids.

Make sure your LO is wearing comfortable shoes that fit well, which may not be the shoes they own. Feet can widen, and even lengthen, with age. Replace tight-fitting socks with loose cotton socks. Wash and dry their feet every day, and dry the areas in between their toes. Slather moisturizer on their clean, dry feet and allow the moisturizer to seep into the skin before putting on shoes and socks.

- For calluses: Gently rub them with a callus file or pumice stone and apply nonmedicated bandages to protect them.
- For dry, cracked heels: Moisturize clean feet.
- For heel pain: Add heel pads or cups to shoes to relieve pressure.
- For toenails: Trim nails straight across the toe's top. If toenails look damaged, bring your LO to see a doctor.

HEARING PROBLEMS

Many elderly people in general have hearing loss, which can exacerbate dementia/AD symptoms; when your LO can't hear, they may be more confused and agitated, causing depression and social withdrawal. The ears pick up environmental cues that help with balance, too, so if they are hard of hearing, your LO is at a greater risk for falling.

It can be hard to tell if hearing loss is an issue, but there are little tells. If you notice that your LO cannot detect high-pitched sounds like a child's voice, or can't follow a conversation on the phone, they may be having hearing issues.

Check your LO's ears for wax buildup, and gently clean them regularly. If the buildup is severe, a doctor can remove the wax with special tools. Some medications, a head injury, or an infection can play a role in temporary hearing loss.

The best way to treat hearing loss is with hearing aids, yet many people do not look into this option because they are afraid of the cost. And rightly so: in the past, good hearing aids cost thousands of dollars and required specialized fittings from a physician. However, in 2017 the federal government passed the Over-The-Counter Hearing Aid Act, which will significantly bring down the price of these devices once it is approved by the FDA.

INFECTIONS/COLDS/COVID/FLU/ALLERGIES

Older people in general are more susceptible to colds and infections because their immune systems are weaker. Infections, colds, allergies, and viruses like the flu or COVID all cause inflammation inside the body and brain, which could make dementia/AD symptoms like confusion and fatigue worse. So it's important to know what your LO is dealing with if they feel sick, especially if they have a virus that could spread to you or other members of your team.

The best way for you and your LO to prevent infections is to practice good hygiene, including frequent hand washing, and keep up with immunizations. You and your LO should be vaccinated for COVID and shingles (if you are over 50), and get a yearly flu shot.

If your LO has seasonal allergies, they may have watery eyes, coughing, sneezing, headache, sore throat, and sometimes a fever. Treat with over-the-counter antihistamines and keep your windows closed at all times. An air purifier is a worthwhile investment that keeps allergens out of indoor air.

It's hard to determine if your LO has a cold or the flu, or even COVID. If your LO has a fever that increases with or without other symptoms for more than 24 hours, take them to see their doctor or arrange for a telehealth consultation.

SKIN ISSUES

Older adults develop a variety of skin conditions. While they have little to do with dementia/AD, they can make life uncomfortable and lead to behavioral consequences. Dry skin, for example, can crack and lead to infections, particularly on the feet. It can also lead to *pruritus*, the most common skin disorder among older people, which is like eczema. It is defined as an unpleasant sensation that provokes the desire to scratch. Your LO should be fully moisturized twice a day to prevent both dry skin and pruritus, and more often if you notice their skin is drier than normal, which can happen in cold climates.

Bedsores, pressure sores, and pressure ulcers are three names for the same ailment, which most often occurs in the late stages of the disease. Sores can develop if your LO is sitting or lying in the same position for too long. In fact, a bedsore can develop in as little as 2 hours. On lighter skin tones, pressure sores look like red patches, and for people with darker skin tones, they appear as patchy skin with a blue or purple tint. The sores often develop over bony areas of the body, like heels, ankles, inner knees, buttocks, hips, spine, elbows, shoulder blades, ears, and the back of the head.

There are four distinct categories of pressure sores; watch carefully for the early signs of skin damage, because if they are left untreated, these sores can become painful and infected.

Category 1: If you touch a discolored patch of skin lightly and it remains discolored, it is likely the earliest sign of a sore. Your LO may also complain that the area is painful, harder or softer than the surrounding skin, or hot. Use pressure-relieving pads, special cushions, or mattresses to prevent pressure ulcers from getting worse, but avoid donut or ring-shaped cushions, which reduce flow to the area. Wash the area with a gentle cleanser and pat dry. Create a moisture barrier with a protective ointment to protect the area from bodily fluids if the sore is near the face, genitals, or upper legs. Avoid positions that put pressure on the existing sore. Do not massage the skin near or on the ulcer.

Category 2: The skin is broken and there may be an open wound, like a scrape or a blister, that can lead to infection. To treat, clean the wound with salt water: do not use hydrogen peroxide or iodine, both of which can further damage the skin. Keep the sore completely covered with a bandage. You can also give your LO a pain reliever, like Tylenol, Motrin, or Aleve.

Category 3: The skin is broken to a deeper level, causing a crater that may reveal the fat cells underneath the skin and can lead to infection. Bring your LO to a doctor immediately.

Category 4: These craters will be deeper and, in extreme cases, can reveal a bone. These sores can cause serious damage to your LO's skin, joints, and tendons and can lead to infection. Bring your LO to a doctor immediately.

To prevent future bedsores:

- Change your LO's position every 15 minutes if they are sitting up, or every 2 hours if they are bedridden, daytime or nighttime.

- Keep your LO's skin clean and well-moisturized.

- Sheepskin products will protect their body where pressure sores typically develop. Place your LO directly onto a sheepskin bed pad or chair cushion. There are also sheepskin slippers, elbow pads, and neck pillows. These products are made of natural fibers that reduce tension on pressure points while maintaining a comfortable and consistent body temperature.

- Use an over-the-counter paste or ointment containing zinc oxide to proactively create a protective barrier around the areas where pressure sores are likely to develop.

- Use extra pillows to support your LO in a variety of positions in bed or if they are in a wheelchair.

Burns

Burns can range from sunburn to an accidental encounter with a hot object, like a stove, a barbecue grill, or even a hot car. There are three main types of burns:

First-degree burns result in a reddening of the outer layer of skin that is often accompanied by pain. A mild sunburn is a typical first-degree burn. An over-the-counter pain reliever like Tylenol or Advil will address inflammation (the reddening), and applying ice or a very cold compress to the burn for about 10 minutes is typically all that is required. Aloe vera cream, petroleum jelly, or antibiotic ointment can be used to cover the burn while it heals and should be applied a few times a day. Do not use household remedies like toothpaste or butter, no matter what you have read on the Internet.

Second-degree burns also have swelling and blistering. A clean, nonstick bandage needs to be applied to cover any broken skin and can be used with aloe vera cream, petroleum jelly, or antibiotic ointment. Change the bandage and ointment daily until the burn has healed. Do not pop any blisters.

Third-degree burns require immediate medical attention because the surface of the skin is broken and possibly numb. Your LO may go into shock and develop pale and clammy skin, weakness, bluish lips and fingernails, and more pronounced confusion. Call 911 or take your LO to the doctor or emergency room. In the meantime, cover the burned area with a clean, cool washcloth or a slightly wet bandage. Submerging a large burn in water can cause a sudden drop in body temperature and lead to hypothermia. Keep the burned area raised above the heart if possible. Depending on the severity, a burn can take weeks to heal. During that time, protect the area from the sun: wear protective clothing and apply sunscreen with an SPF of 30 or higher. This will help minimize scarring, especially if your LO has a dark skin tone.

Prevent Future Burns

- Keep a fire extinguisher handy.
- Keep blankets in your car and cover the seats if you will be parked in direct sun.
- Replace the batteries in smoke detectors and carbon monoxide detectors once a year.
- Separate electrical appliances from water sources and unplug them when they're not in use.
- Set a firm rule for your LO: no smoking in bed or without supervision.
- Set the water heater to under 120 degrees, and always check the temperature of the shower water before bathing your LO.
- Turn the handles of pots and pans toward the back of the stove, keeping them farther away from your LO.

SLEEP ISSUES

One health issue almost all people with dementia/AD face is disrupted sleep. Poor sleep exacerbates cognitive decline for both patients and caregivers. As we get older, some people have a harder time falling asleep or wake up more often in the middle of the night.

Others wake up earlier in the morning or sleep later, especially after a restless night. The transition between sleep and waking up can become more abrupt as well.

These are all normal sleep disturbances that occur as we age. Yet with dementia/AD, these nighttime problems can be more extreme. What I've seen in my nursing practice corroborates with the Mayo Clinic's research: sleep disturbances tend to get worse as dementia/AD progresses, and getting the right amount of sleep each night is key to your LO's overall success during the day.[1] Likewise, I've found that people with dementia/AD who sleep better at night are in a better mood the next day; are in better overall health; and have an easier time making decisions, solving problems, controlling their emotions, and coping with change. These are all the factors you want to maintain as the disease progresses.

You may find that your LO is excessively tired on some days, leading to long daytime naps. These can be followed by insomnia episodes with trouble falling asleep and staying asleep, early-morning awakenings, and oversleeping. You may be thinking, *What's the big deal if my husband sleeps during the day?* Well, there are two reasons to get your LO on a sleep schedule. First, poor sleep—including getting too much—will affect their mood and their memory. If they aren't sleeping well, they can't think well. What's more, when your LO sleeps at night, so will you. One of the clearest causes of caregiver stress and burnout is poor sleep, so we want to do everything we can to avoid that.

The best way to get your LO to sleep at the right time is to set up a schedule for sleep and include it in your Family Care Plan. The goal is to have your LO in bed and sleeping for 7 to 8 hours each night. No more, no less.

If your LO is having sleeping issues, let's figure out why and swap habits that aren't working for new ones that promote better sleep. All the reasons for sleep disruption listed in Chapter 3 as to why you may be having a hard time sleeping apply to your LO: acid reflux caused by eating too late, dehydration, sleeping with a pet, or snoring/sleep apnea. Making small adjustments, such as keeping a non-breakable cup of water near the bed (which is why I love the "mini fridge as bedside table" idea, to keep water bottles handy), moving the dog to another room, or having dinner earlier, will help your LO get a better night's sleep.

Then take the following aspects of their day into account:

- Check medications; a frequent side effect of many medications is sleep disturbance. Talk to your LO's doctor if you think their meds are interfering, and see if they can switch their prescription to another that may be better tolerated. Specifically, some antidepressants, such as Wellbutrin and Effexor XR, can lead to insomnia. Aricept is often prescribed for people with dementia/ AD in the early stages, because it is thought to improve cognitive and behavioral symptoms, but it also can cause insomnia.

- Did they spend a large chunk of the day in a dark room? The average adult spends at least 60 minutes a day in bright sunlight, but for people with dementia/AD, it can be as little as 30 minutes. Make sure that your inside rooms are bright for most of the day, and get outside for at least an hour if weather permits.

- Is the bedroom too noisy, too light, or too warm? Bedrooms need to be "just right": dark, quiet, and cool. Turn down the thermostat or switch out the blankets so your LO is cooler. If one of you sleeps "hot" and the other sleeps "cold," adjust the temperature/bedding to the cooler side and add another layer to the other person's bedding.

- Review their day; were they mentally or physically exhausted at the end of the day, or did they have a day that was highly disorientating and off the care plan? Change in general can affect sleep.

- Too little exercise? You and your LO need 30 minutes of exercise every day, as long as they are able to move on their own. That's why the sample Family Care Plans in Chapter 2 include a workout every day.

- Too much coffee? Swap in decaf after 3:00 p.m.

- Were they acting out while dreaming? People with Lewy body dementia often experience hallucinations accompanied by body movements, which can awaken them.

- What stage of dementia/AD are they in? As the disease progresses, sleep problems become more pronounced.

There are a handful of behavioral fixes to try:

- Limit daytime naps or rest periods to 30 minutes each.

- No more bedtime snacks! While some people say it helps them sleep to nosh before bed, it messes with your circadian rhythm, which is the way your body is calibrated to do certain activities at certain times of the day. Your body is not meant to digest food during sleep.

- Avoid stimulation, such as violent TV shows, and blue light devices, such as televisions, cell phones, and computer screens, before bedtime.

- Establish a relaxing bedtime routine and make it part of your care plan. Before your LO gets into pajamas, I recommend using this time for their daily shower because it is so relaxing. Then stick with the activities that they have always done after dinner, as long as they are not overstimulating. You may have to replace exciting television shows with something calmer, like soothing music, conversation, or reading to your LO.

- If your LO wakes up during the night, stay calm and find out what they need. It's possible that they are in pain or dehydrated or need to use the bathroom. Attend to their needs with as little light as possible. Then gently remind them it's nighttime and put them back into bed.

- Your LO may need to pace during the night. If this happens, don't restrain them; allow it under your supervision for a few minutes and then guide them back to bed.

Finally, consider the following treatments to promote a better night's sleep. Discuss all of these with your LO's doctor before you implement them; try only one at a time for at least a week, and record your findings in your Daily Observation:

- Is your LO being treated for other conditions that affect sleep? Depression, anxiety, sleep apnea, and restless leg syndrome are the most common culprits.

- Change the time your LO takes medication; administering medications before dinnertime often helps people with dementia/AD get a better night's sleep.

- Try bright light therapy in the evening, which may help your LO reset their sleep patterns. A light therapy box exposes their eyes to intense but safe amounts of light for a specific length of time. Side effects like eye irritation and dryness, headache, nausea, and dry skin can be alleviated if you begin the therapy slowly, for just a few minutes at a time, giving the body time to get used to it. Using a humidifier at the same time can help with dryness.

- Consider melatonin. Melatonin can be bought over the counter as a supplement, or in a prescription version called ramelteon, which is thought to last longer.

- Consider magnesium supplements. Older people have less available magnesium, and it is thought that supplementing can help people with dementia/AD increase sleep time. You can also try adding foods high in magnesium into their diet, like nuts (see page 246 for more food suggestions).

- Antihistamines like Benadryl and Tylenol PM can help your LO fall asleep and stay asleep but can also lead to daytime drowsiness.

- Prescription sleep aids such as Valium, Xanax, Ambien, and suvorexant are effective sleep medications, but they also increase the risk of falls and confusion among people with dementia/AD. This is why these medications aren't typically recommended. If these medications are prescribed, they should only be used on occasion, or for short periods of time until a regular sleep pattern is established.

- "Off-label" medications can help; for example, your doctor may prescribe antidepressants like trazodone, Remeron, or Sinequan for sleep purposes. Antipsychotic medications like Perseris can also help.

Is It Fatigue or Lethargy?

Fatigue, lethargy, and indecisiveness are all signs of dementia/AD. In the earlier stages, some people experience dementia fatigue, which is an overwhelming decrease in energy, and later, many people with dementia/AD sleep soundly during the day and night.

However, if your LO's sleep patterns have changed significantly from their typical behavior, they may not be getting the right balance of key vitamins in their diet. Low levels of vitamin D, iron, magnesium, or potassium can cause fatigue and confusion. A vitamin B_{12} deficiency may lead to numbness in the hands and feet. Your LO's doctor can perform a quick blood test to identify a deficiency and may recommend supplements to get their levels up. See the suggestions in Chapter 9 for foods that are high in these nutrients.

URINARY TRACT INFECTIONS (UTIs)

Painful urination, frequent urination, an ongoing urge to urinate, pelvic-area pain, fever, chills, and urine with a strong odor are all signs of this type of bacterial infection. It occurs most commonly in women, but men experience them as well. Aside from physical pain, they can cause increased confusion for people with dementia/AD, as well as incontinence, agitation, decreased mobility, and loss of appetite. In fact, it's one of the primary causes of disruptive behaviors, likely because they are in so much pain but can't communicate what's bothering them. If left untreated, this infection can spread to the kidneys and cause back pain, nausea, and vomiting. If it enters the bloodstream, it can be life-threatening.

Your LO's doctor can confirm a UTI with a simple urine test, and there are home tests as well. If the results are positive, your doctor will prescribe antibiotics. Your LO should drink at least six to eight 8-ounce water bottles every day, and more if they need to flush out the bacteria. You can administer over-the-counter pain relievers to ease the burning sensation. Tylenol and Advil may help, but the best choice is a product made especially for this condition, called AZO.

To prevent UTIs from recurring, your LO needs to be reminded to clean themselves well after using the bathroom, and to change their disposable underwear. Both should be addressed every 2 hours. And make sure they are drinking plenty of water throughout the day to prevent these infections from taking hold.

VISION PROBLEMS

Aside from the typical problems of aging eyes, dementia/AD can cause changes to the way your LO sees and how the brain processes visual information. First, your LO's field of vision can narrow: normal peripheral vision is about twenty feet, but your LO's may be limited to around a foot in front and to the sides of their face. That's a significant difference. What's more, their brain, in an effort to understand visual information, often shuts off the input coming from one eye, which can lead to a loss of depth perception or the ability to discern colors. That means your LO will have a harder time finding and picking up items, turning on and off lights, and even walking.

Your LO may also experience *reduced gaze*, which is a noted dementia/AD symptom. If this occurs, your LO will have less ability to move their eyes and track objects, and instead look like they are staring into space.

Unfortunately, there isn't a real fix for these problems. However, it's still important to record them, because they may help explain unusual behaviors that seem to "come out of nowhere." Your LO should continue to have their eyes checked annually so that other issues that can be addressed, like glaucoma, cataracts, and macular degeneration, are kept in check.

PREPARING TO SEE A DOCTOR

Every time your LO needs to see a doctor, you should accompany them. This is true for both in-person appointments and telehealth visits. Don't outsource this task to another member of your team; as the primary caregiver, you need firsthand information on how your LO is progressing through this and any other disease. Bring the healthcare proxy that we discussed in Chapter 2 to any appointment.

Prepare yourself for the visit beforehand. Review your binder and your Daily Observations so that you can accurately describe what's going on. Write down your thoughts on a separate piece of paper, including any concerns or questions. Bringing written notes will help you remember them and may come in handy if your LO refuses to let you into the examination room. Also, bring your binder to show the doctor any trends that you have noticed, and remind them of any medications prescribed by other doctors they may not be aware of.

Your LO may also require lab work, which they may order while you are in the office, so they won't be able to analyze the results while you're there. Instead, call the doctor's office in advance and request to do the lab work beforehand. That way they will have all the information they need at the appointment. Ask if the doctor has all the medical records from any other specialist your LO is seeing. If they don't, arrange for them to be sent over; do not leave this task to the doctor's staff, and if you do, follow up again before your visit.

Then prepare your LO. Going to a doctor can produce anxiety, which is why I do not recommend telling them too far ahead of time. When you get to the office, use direct communication to tell your LO in a calm way, using their name, what to expect, and reassure them that you will not leave them.

Ideally, you will be in the room during the examination. Your role is to be the moderator, as you will have a better understanding of what's going on with your LO than the doctor. You also have to act as your LO's advocate, so take notes in the binder during your visit. Use your phone to record the conversation so you can review it again when you get home.

If your LO refuses to let you into the examination room, give the piece of paper with your list of concerns to the receptionist, and ask them to give it to the doctor. Then, when your LO's exam is over, have a separate conversation with the doctor before you leave the office.

Last, always ask the doctor if your LO is a candidate for any clinical studies or trials related to dementia/AD. This opens the door to have a conversation about the latest research. If your doctor doesn't know how to enroll your LO, you haven't found the best doctor. Find another doctor who is better informed, or go to the Alzheimer's Association website at www.alz.org/TrialMatch to learn more.

If Your LO Is Afraid to See a Doctor

Many people avoid medical care, for a variety of reasons. Some believe that doctors do not have their best interests at heart, and honestly, this is understandable, especially for minority communities. However, we can't let the practices of the past influence the present or your LO's future. Your LO absolutely needs to see a physician regularly, so it's up to you to help them get the care they deserve and are comfortable with. If you can find a doctor that is the same race or gender as your LO, they may feel more confident that they are receiving the right level of care.

You will also have to act as a well-informed advocate. Educate yourself about your LO's health status before you walk into the doctor's office, and be prepared to communicate clearly. Then remind your LO that as their caregiver, you are there to make sure that nothing bad happens to them.

EVERYTHING YOU NEED TO KNOW ABOUT DEMENTIA/AD MEDICATIONS

Certain medications that are prescribed to treat dementia/AD symptoms are effective in resolving pain and behavioral issues. Unfortunately, despite optimistic headlines every once in a while, including the 2021 FDA approval for Aduhelm, an intravenous medication that may delay mild cognitive decline, there is no medication that reverses memory loss and loss of cognitive function.

Discuss each of these with your LO's doctor so that you understand their pros and cons, and see if they will interact with any other medications your LO may already be taking.

Cognitive stabilizers: Memantine (Namenda) is used to treat moderate to severe dementia/AD. It does not cure AD, but it may improve memory, awareness, and the ability to perform daily functions. Cholinesterase inhibitors are another category of drugs thought to do the same, and they include donepezil (Aricept), galantamine (Razadyne), and rivastigmine (Exelon). Each may help lessen or stabilize cognitive function, although none can reverse skills that have been lost.

Antidepressants: Sertraline (Zoloft), citalopram (Celexa), mirtazapine (Remeron), and trazodone (Desyrel, Oleptro) are widely prescribed for people with dementia who develop depression. Some are also used as sleep aids.

Antipsychotics: Medicines that treat paranoia and confusion, called neuroleptics or antipsychotics, include aripiprazole (Abilify), haloperidol (Haldol), olanzapine (Zyprexa), quetiapine (Seroquel), risperidone (Risperdal), and ziprasidone (Geodon). Some are also used as sleep aids.

Mood stabilizers: These drugs address aggression and irritability. The most frequently prescribed are sodium valproate (Depakote) and carbamazepine (Tegretol).

Stimulants: Methylphenidate (Ritalin, Concerta) is prescribed for apathy or treatment-resistant depression.

Guided medical cannabis: Medical research is beginning to look at cannabis options as effective treatment solutions for people with dementia/AD, and doctors are taking note. In states where it is legal, recreational and medical cannabis products can be used as mood stabilizers and sleep aids. If your doctor is not well-versed in medical

cannabis use, you can find a telehealth physician consultant at www
.justanswer.com, www.ezdoctor.com, and www.amwell.com.

ADMINISTERING MEDICATION

If your LO has a prescription regimen, a calendared pillbox that you
can set up for two weeks or a month at a time ensures that they have
taken their medication each day. Pharmacies like CVS can also take
all of your LO's prescriptions and sort them into daily pill packets,
which can be dated.

Set an alarm on your cell phone to administer the medication at
the right time each day, per the doctor's instructions on the label.
There are also medication reminder apps for your smartphone; even
home assistants like Alexa can be programmed to give prompts.

Become familiar with the likely side effects of each medication,
which is provided when you pick up the prescription. Don't throw it
out; read it and make notes so that you know what to expect. Keep a
medication chart in your binder so that you can quickly reference
what your LO is taking and the current dosages. Then, when you are
doing your Daily Observation, see if your LO is reacting to their medication. Were they more agitated than usual because you introduced
a new drug? Or were they more sedated? Some people can take as long
as six months to adjust to new prescriptions.

CHAPTER 9

Navigating Mealtime

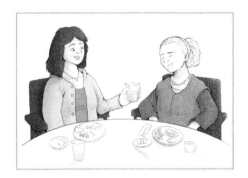

Though it sounds hard to believe, one of the trickiest parts of care-giving for someone with dementia/AD is making sure that they eat well, and eat enough, every day. We take eating for granted because it seems to come so naturally: we feel hungry, we search for food, we prepare it, and then we eat it. Now, it's likely that your LO will have difficulty with each part of the process.

Even in the earliest stages your LO may not feel as hungry as they used to. And when they are hungry, they can be confused by the choices in the refrigerator: what foods are for each meal, or what foods go together (peanut butter and jelly versus peanut butter and mustard). Cooking becomes harder and dangerous. And to make matters more complicated, when it comes to dementia/AD, every person is different. So while some people in the early stages forget how to cook, others forget that food needs to be defrosted before cooking, or that dessert is eaten after a meal, not before.

I was hired to care for Alice, who had early-stage AD. Her family was concerned because she was losing weight. When I got there, I realized that she had not eaten properly for weeks and had lost about ten pounds. She had plenty of food in the house; she just wasn't feeling hungry and didn't remember that she hadn't eaten. I created a meal chart, put it in the kitchen, and added a sticker after each meal. In just a few weeks, Alice gained back all the weight she lost and had a process she could follow to ensure that she wouldn't skip meals again.

As the disease progresses into the moderate stages your LO may struggle with these same problems, and new ones may emerge. They may not recognize what is on their plate or remember how to use silverware. If they are physically uncomfortable, depressed, or tired, they may not be able to focus on finishing an entire meal. I have seen situations in which a person with moderate dementia/AD stopped eating their favorite foods and started asking for something entirely unexpected. Sometimes they develop a taste for spicy foods or foods with a particular texture or crunch. Or they may remember a favorite treat from their youth. I've also noticed that they like to add more salt or sweeteners (sometimes way too much); as their ability to taste and smell diminishes, food in general doesn't taste as good, and they are trying to amplify the flavors—or they forgot they added it already. In general, they develop a sweet tooth, even if they didn't crave desserts before.

In the late stages your LO may forget how to chew and swallow. As they become increasingly nonverbal, they may act out when they are frustrated about their food, or if they are in pain when they are eating. This is when you will have to get really creative, so read on. This chapter will provide everything you need to know to ensure that your LO is eating and thriving.

STRATEGIES FOR MEALTIME

Let's start by talking strategy: the goal is to get your LO to eat first on their own, and later, with your assistance. In the early stages, your LO will be able to feed themselves, although you may have to remind them that it is mealtime, and they may need help with cooking and cleaning up. Meal planning and prep can be activities that you and your LO do together, although I don't advise making the actual cooking the focus. It's just too risky for your LO to be around sharp knives or hot surfaces.

Well into the moderate stages your LO will likely be able to let you know which foods agree with them, which ones they look forward to, and how they like them prepared. However, they may need help remembering when to eat, how to eat, and how to use utensils. It's very likely that during this middle stage you will have to cut up your LO's food into bite-sized pieces before you present it to them.

An occupational therapist on your team can also make great recommendations. They may suggest specific types of tableware that aren't sharp, are easy to hold, and will not create a mess. For instance, introduce sippy cups that are meant for toddlers, with slanted sides, handles, and a lip. You can find ones for either hot or cold beverages. I particularly like the Reflo Smart Cup, because it looks like an adult cup but has a barrier inside so that you can't fill it completely, and your LO can use it without a straw (straws are not ideal for those with dementia/AD, as they actually can impede swallowing).

In the later stages, you may need to start pureeing cooked foods, which are easy to eat and packed with nutrition. The need for this switch will be evident if your LO is struggling with chewing or swallowing, as pureed foods will lower the risk of choking. A pureed diet consists of foods that are blended, whipped, or mashed and includes fruits and vegetables, chicken and fish, ground meats, milkshakes, pudding, and soups. High-calorie drinks and protein shakes are also good options, as are stewed, boiled, or mashed fruits and vegetables and overcooked rice and pasta. You may think that a quick fix to prepare pureed foods is to start with baby food, but I don't recommend it. Adults need more nutrients than what is formulated for babies, and a couple of jars per meal is not going to sustain them.

MAKE MEALS EASY

The following mealtime tips can be introduced whenever you see fit:

- At each meal, offer just one food at a time—for example, a protein, then a vegetable, then rice—instead of presenting a "balanced" plate that has too many foods on it. Start with small portions; you can always give them more food.

- Breakfast should be the largest meal of the day, as your LO will probably be hungry when they wake up. Use this meal to ensure that they have enough calories to sustain them for the entire day if later meals aren't as successful.

- Eat with your LO; they will mirror your movements and eat more of the food that's on their plate.

- Offer soft finger foods for snacks as well as whole meals: think cheese, fresh berries, and small, soft sandwiches.

- Hot meals should be delivered warm, not piping-hot. Your LO may not be able to judge food temperature and can easily burn their mouth.

Tips for Getting Your LO to Swallow

In the late stages, your LO may lose the ability to swallow foods and medications. Poor swallowing is a serious problem because it can lead to weight loss, choking, or pulling foods or liquids directly into the lungs, which can cause pneumonia. Try these swallowing tips:

- Cut all soft foods into small pieces.
- Once your LO has taken a bite, gently stroke their neck in a downward motion and say the word "swallow." This trick is useful for foods as well as medications.
- Offer soft foods at every meal, such as eggs, yogurt, soups, cottage cheese, or tuna fish.
- Serve beverages at various safe temperatures to see which are easiest to drink.
- Stick to less viscous liquids. Milk can catch in the throat.
- Straws can make swallowing problems worse. Have your LO take small sips from a cup.
- Switch pill medications to a liquid form, or find out if the pills can be crushed into soft foods or drinks.
- Your LO should be sitting upright for every meal and should stay seated for at least 20 minutes afterward, even when they are bedridden.

If your LO is still having difficulty, be proactive and talk to their doctor about hiring a speech/language pathologist. Say something like, *"I've been observing this for a week. I just weighed my loved one. I've been monitoring their weight. They're not eating all their food, so I need to take them for an evaluation, maybe with a speech/language pathologist."*

- If your LO wears dentures, make sure that they are well-fitting, which will make chewing easier.

- Keep dangerous prep tools away from your LO's reach. Empty the dishwasher and put away dishes and silverware while your LO is sleeping.

- Meals should be a time for eating and conversation only. Turn off the TV or other distractions, like music, *unless* you find that these background noises are soothing for your LO.

- Meals will take longer to complete. Sometimes your LO may need a break in the middle of a meal. Try again a little later; they may still be hungry.

- Mealtime may get messy. Try not to stress about it; you can always clean up afterward. Use plastic place mats or tablecloths that are easily wiped down.

- Raw, hard vegetables can pose a problem; blanch raw vegetables to make them softer and still provide a crunch.

- Serve meals at the same time each day as part of a routine, which will make sticking to your care plan easier.

- Offer snacks throughout the day to make sure that they are getting enough calories. However, nibbling all day long can make mealtimes less successful. Find a balance with light snacks instead of heavy ones.

THE BEST FOODS FOR YOU AND YOUR LO

Your LO can and should eat all of the foods that they enjoy. They will likely lose weight during this disease. As the caregiver, you need to keep them well fed and provide the calories they need to energize their brain and body. That doesn't mean they should eat processed junk food or ice cream for every meal, but it's fair to say they can have dessert every day. In short, the best foods for your LO will be the ones they love, prepared the way they like them.

As much as I wish it were true, though, you will not benefit from partaking in this liberal attitude toward food. In order to provide the best care, you need to be at your best, which means focusing on foods that are nutrient-dense, which will improve your cardiovascular health, help you manage your weight, and even promote better sleep. If you recognize that you could be eating healthier, start with the standard Mediterranean diet, which many doctors recommend for lowering inflammation and which can help prevent and manage heart disease and diabetes. While there are no magic foods that reverse or prevent dementia/AD, lowering inflammation can maintain cognitive status and slow down decline. Since these foods are healthy choices anyway, you don't have much to lose by focusing on them for both you and your LO and eating them in place of foods that we know are bad for us, like those filled with simple sugars and unhealthy fats.

The basic rules for the Mediterranean diet focus on complex carbohydrates that are whole foods (fruits, vegetables and grains); proteins like eggs, fish, meat, and poultry; and monounsaturated fats that are liquid or soft at room temperature, like olive oil. My favorite Mediterranean diet foods include the following. Choose from this list when you are planning each meal for you and your LO:

- Avocado
- Beans
- Berries
- Chicken
- Coconut oil
- Dairy: whole-milk products including yogurt and cheese

- Eggs
- High-fiber bran cereal
- Leafy green vegetables
- Mild spices like turmeric/curcumin
- Nuts and seeds (chopped to prevent choking)
- Olives
- Omega-3 fatty acid foods like salmon
- Whole grains (instead of white bread products)

Foods High in Important Nutrients

Include the following foods every day. These are naturally high in the vitamins your LO needs:

- To increase vitamins D and B12: fortified milk products, fortified breakfast cereals, fortified tofu, fresh fish, eggs
- To increase iron: lentils, spinach, soybeans/tofu, chickpeas, apricots, cashews, almonds, quinoa, red meats/liver
- To increase magnesium: avocado, nuts, tofu, seeds, whole grains, fatty fish (salmon), bananas, leafy greens, okra, potatoes (with the skin)
- To increase potassium: bananas, oranges, cantaloupe, honeydew, apricots, grapefruit, green vegetables, potatoes, yams

---

A WEEKLY MEAL PLAN

I always prepare foods I know that my patients like, and I make sure there is variety. Use the chart on pages 248–249 as a baseline; it's my go-to for nutritious meals for people in the early and moderate stages.

These suggestions incorporate the preceding food lists and are meant to help your LO avoid both constipation and urinary tract infections. A protein shake can always be added as an additional snack if your LO is losing weight. And don't forget to give your LO plenty of water throughout the day.

LATE-STAGE DIETARY CHANGES

In the late stages, you will end up pureeing your LO's food. First, cut raw foods into small pieces, removing seeds, pits, skins, or other inedible parts before cooking. Then boil or bake the food until it is as soft as possible, and mash by hand. You can also use a food processor or blender; look for one that crushes ice and other hard foods, like carrots. Add small amounts of water or broth to help achieve the desired consistency. The more water added, the thinner the consistency will be. Finally, season with salt, sugar, or honey.

THE TRUTH ABOUT SUPPLEMENTS

The last piece of the nutrition puzzle is supplements. Sometimes, even when you are trying your best, your LO may not be getting the vitamins they need. Supplements can make getting the right nutrition easier. Based on your LO's lab work, their doctor may tell you that your LO is deficient in vitamins and/or minerals. However, not all supplements are regulated by the FDA, and it's impossible to know whether what you are paying for is what you are getting. My advice is to stick with getting your nutrients from foods whenever possible, and use supplements as a last resort.

SAMPLE

	Monday	Tuesday	Wednesday
Breakfast	Flavored yogurt Banana slices Bran muffin Coffee	Fried eggs Whole-grain toast Cranberry juice Coffee	French toast Sausage patties Coffee
Snack	Fresh fruit in season	Fresh fruit in season	Fresh fruit in season
Lunch	Broiled chicken Avocado slices	Vegetable stir-fry with rice	Grilled cheese sandwich Steamed broccoli
Snack	Chocolate pudding	Oatmeal cookies	Apple crisp
Dinner	Rice and beans Green salad with cucumbers and peppers	Pan-fried salmon fillet Baked butternut squash	Turkey meatloaf Quinoa Caesar salad
Snack	Cheese and crackers	Bran cereal and milk	Hummus and celery

MEAL

WEEKLY

Thursday	Friday	Saturday	Sunday
Oatmeal with raisins Cranberry juice Coffee	Scrambled eggs with bacon Whole-grain toast Coffee	Melon slices Cottage cheese Cranberry juice Coffee	Cheese omelet ½ grapefruit Whole-grain toast Coffee
Fresh fruit in season	Fresh fruit in season	Fresh fruit in season	Fresh fruit in season
Hamburger Baked polenta fries	Eggplant Parmesan Green salad with tomatoes Dinner roll	Tuna fish with dried cranberries over salad greens	Chicken salad Baby carrots and spinach dip
Rice pudding	Lemon bars	Ice cream sundae	Slice of pie
Roast chicken Dried apricots Roasted cauliflower	Slow cooker pulled pork sandwich Coleslaw	Chicken Parmesan Roasted brussels sprouts	LO's favorite dinner
Peanut butter and apple slices	Bran cereal and milk	Granola bar	Chex mix

PLAN

What's more, there is little research that shows that any supplement helps slow the progression of the disease. In fact, in 2019 the Global Council on Brain Health released an official document stating unequivocally that they don't. So no matter what you have seen on television, save your money, unless the physician specifically recommends a supplement to fill a nutritional need.

INVESTIGATE FOOD SERVICES YOUR COMMUNITY OFFERS

The best tip of all is to enroll your LO in a local Meals on Wheels program to receive free, or low-cost daily meals. Meals on Wheels operates more than five thousand independently run programs that are funded by federal and state governments and private donors. The number of meals your LO will receive is determined by how well funded the branch is in your community. Your LO may get a meal and a snack, or two full meals.

Anyone over age 60, no matter how much money they have, qualifies for Meals on Wheels, which is why I highly recommend that you use it. It takes preparing at least one meal a day off your responsibility list. When I signed up my aunt, she received two meals a day and snacks, delivered to her door, so the only meal I needed to prepare was breakfast. Even if your LO doesn't eat every meal, at least you know that if the day is not going perfectly, you can supplement the meal you are making with this food.

There is an application process and, in some locations, a waiting list. For more information, contact your local program or visit the national website at www.mealsonwheelsamerica.org.

CHAPTER 10

Coordinating Respite Care

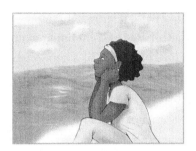

You already know that even the most loving caregivers need a break. As we've discussed, the best way to ensure that you get these breaks consistently is to use your team to provide coverage, and schedule that coverage into the Family Care Plan. However, there will be times when your team isn't available, or your need for coverage extends beyond their capabilities. Maybe you want to take a vacation, you develop an infectious illness, or you just don't feel well. This type of coverage is referred to as *respite care*.

Full-day respite care can be arranged through an adult daycare center, which may be a free benefit from your community or carry a fee. To make the most of this option, your LO should be acclimated to this service as early as possible so that they can adapt to the center's routines. These centers work particularly well for people in the earliest stages of the disease and are less useful later, because many require that you stay with your LO (which means they're not a great choice if you are looking to take a day off). The best adult daycare centers offer a stimulating social environment, mental and physical activities, emergency and ongoing health services (like PT or OT), meals or snacks, assistance with ADLs, and even transportation. Look for one that specifically caters to people with dementia/AD. They are typically open Monday through Friday.

Another option for daily coverage is to have someone come to the home or bring your LO to their home. This home health aide could be a volunteer from a faith-based or community nonprofit organization, or a trained professional organized by a home care business. You may be able to arrange for half-day, full-day, overnight, or longer coverage. Make sure whoever you bring in can handle the specific challenges facing your LO. They are not in any way a replacement for your care, but they should be warm, friendly, and trustworthy.

If you need more than a few days off, a short-term residential program at a group home, personal care residence, or nursing home may be ideal. Many of these facilities provide coverage for a week or two, and they may be covered by insurance. They offer peace of mind when you take a vacation, fall ill, or just need time for yourself. What's more, they offer the opportunity to explore a more permanent living situation. Be prepared for both positive and negative reactions. Some caregivers may believe that their LO would get superior care in this environment for a longer stay in the future. Others may see why the commitment to providing home care is worth the effort.

BEFORE THE FIRST DROP-OFF: DO YOUR HOMEWORK

Even though you are looking for a short-term solution, you need to be diligent as you investigate respite care options. Your LO needs to be completely supervised in a safe and comfortable environment that not only meets their needs but is committed to people with dementia/AD. Home health aides who come to your home should be personally interviewed beforehand and be able to address all of the ADLs and clearly communicate with you and your LO. If they are coming more often than once a week, they should also tidy the LO's immediate environment; they don't clean the whole home, but they can straighten up anything related to your LO's care. They will also follow your Family Care Plan, and you will be in charge of managing them.

For respite care outside the home, you'll need to do even more research. The best place to start is online; look at both the individual facility's websites as well as rating organizations that report to each state's government. Whether you are looking into adult daycare centers or nursing homes, see how they are rated and what services they provide. The Medicare website is an excellent place to start: Google "[your state] nursing home report card" to uncover any reports that your state has filed regarding elder abuse, mismanagement, disregarding policies and guidelines, and annual reviews. When it comes to nursing homes, the Medicare website does much of the hard work for you; it allows you to compare the quality of care for nursing homes in your area. Next, match your research to recommendations from your team; ask your friends, extended family, doctors, PT and OT, social worker, clergy, and geriatric case managers which facilities they have seen firsthand.

Then visit the facility. Drop in during the day, as close to lunchtime as possible, and ask if you can take a tour. See how the staff is treating the clients, the overall cleanliness of the facility, and what meals look like. Be sure to ask the following questions, and make sure you are on board with the answers you receive:

- How much does this cost, and what does Medicare/Medicaid cover?

- Are there additional costs?
- Is all of the equipment Medicaid-certified?
- Can I attend a residents' council meeting? (This question is for residential facilities. If the answer is no, this place is not for your LO.)
- What special accommodations do you have for clients with dementia/AD?
- How do you handle medical emergencies?
- Who is available during the overnight hours (if applicable)?
- How frequently can I get a report on how my LO is doing?
- Can you accommodate my LO's special needs?

The Difficulties of Letting Go

Assuming that you are comfortable with your findings, you should feel confident that your LO is in good hands for the duration of their stay. That doesn't mean that you will be happy with your decision. You may experience a wide range of emotions when you leave your LO in someone else's care for the first time. You may feel like you are abandoning them, or feel guilty that you are going to do something for yourself. You may even feel guilty that you feel relieved. As I've said, you are entitled to all of your emotions. However, if your feelings are standing in the way of getting the break you need, talk to a friend or therapist who can help you sort through them.

THE UNSPOKEN OPTION:
TRANSITIONING TO A RESIDENTIAL FACILITY

As much as you want to avoid this scenario, there may come a time when your LO needs to be moved out of the home. It's more common than you think; according to the Alzheimer's Association, more than 50 percent of residents in nursing homes have some form of dementia, and 67 percent of dementia-related deaths occur in nursing homes.[1] Two-thirds of this population spend their final days in nursing homes, regardless of the quality of care they received beforehand. To me, this demonstrates how challenging caregiving can be, even with the best of intentions and outcomes. Just because you have to consider a change doesn't mean that you didn't do your best or that it is in any way your fault.

I believe that when caregiving requires more than one caregiver daily, or a sudden trauma (like a fall, stroke, or heart attack) lands your LO in a hospital and a return to home is no longer possible, or when caregiving is taking a significant toll on your health, it's time to pursue other options. Having a plan in advance for when these scenarios arise can make all the difference in your ability to accept this transition, as well as your LO's.

So let's be proactive and think about the unthinkable. Talk about this possibility with your LO as early as possible: having a plan, rather than springing a move on them, is the most loving thing you can do. Write down everyone's thoughts and store them with your most important documents. Having this difficult conversation early will make the transition easier if you ever have to do it.

UNDERSTANDING FULL-TIME RESIDENTIAL OPTIONS

Not every senior housing option is acceptable for someone with dementia. Government-subsidized senior housing is nothing more than inexpensive independent living, and assisted living facilities basically offer what you have been providing all along (and most of the time people with dementia/AD are not accepted because these people require full-time supervision).

However, some eldercare facilities are suitable for someone with dementia/AD at a variety of stages:

A skilled nursing inpatient facility, or nursing home: Large or small, these are institutionalized facilities in that they provide a standard of practices. They can be owned and run by the private sector; by religious, ethnic, fraternal, or professional organizations; or town, city, or state governments. They typically provide residents with a bed, meals, rehabilitation services (PT, OT), medical care, and, most importantly, 24/7 supervision by skilled professionals. Look for a facility that has a separate dementia/AD wing or memory care unit and also offers hospice care. These will have a higher staff-to-resident ratio, as much as 1:4. Research them the same way you would research respite care but with one exception: factor in location! Choose a facility and that is easy for you to visit and that meets all safety requirements.

Board and care: Also referred to as a *personal care home*, this option offers services to a small group of people in a home setting, with 24/7 supervision. Your LO may have to share a bedroom or a bathroom. These group homes function in much the same way that you were providing caregiving: they have daily activities, assist with doctor appointments, and provide meals. Staff-to-resident ratios are higher than at a typical nursing home, which means that your LO may receive better care overall. These facilities are licensed and regulated by each state, and the cost may be covered by both private insurance and Medicaid. Be aware that the staff training regulations are different than what is required at a skilled nursing home.

The most noticeable difference between board and care and a skilled nursing home is that you would still be involved in your LO's care as an integral part of their team. You may be responsible for taking them to their doctor and all necessary appointments; board and care is more a housing change than anything else.

TIMING IS EVERYTHING

The best nursing homes and board and care options are often filled to capacity. Do not wait until your LO is in crisis or needs to be transferred to a facility to start doing your research. Many places keep waiting lists; it doesn't hurt to register your LO long before you think a move is necessary.

For both nursing home and board and care facilities, your LO will be interviewed before placement. In some instances, they will not qualify for certain facilities. My friend Rob's grandmother was cared for by full-time home healthcare aides, and when she was in the later stages of the disease, he decided to investigate memory care centers. There were terrific options that were close to his home, and he thought that she might receive better care. However, his grandmother failed the interview. She couldn't participate in any of the activities, and the administrator felt that she wasn't a good fit for any facility that focused solely on dementia/AD. The family was left with a choice: a traditional nursing home or continued home care. They decided that her needs would best be met at home.

There are many reasons why your LO may not be a good fit. My colleague Donald's father was told that he was no longer a fit for the nursing home that he was living in. His father could no longer eat solid foods and was placed on an all-liquid diet. Donald learned that in some states, nursing homes need special licenses to provide that kind of care, and the facility he was living in didn't have that license. Donald ended up moving his father from Florida to live closer to him in New York. He was able to move into a new apartment with skilled nursing provided by a local PACE program (see Chapter 2).

If your LO is a good fit and you find the right place for them, there are best practices for visiting. Know the visiting hours for the facility; most run between 10:00 a.m. and 8:00 p.m. Always check in with the staff whenever you come: the more you are involved, the better the care will be. There are typically three shifts of staffing for round-the-clock care: stagger your visits so that you can meet each staff rotation and evaluate how they treat your LO. If you plan your visits around mealtimes, you can help the staff by feeding your LO yourself, and observe the socialization opportunities and routines of the facility.

Moving-Day Tips

- Meet family members of other residents beforehand; this is a good way to find out what's really going on inside the nursing home.
- Sew nametags into all clothing items.
- Pack much-loved home furnishing items and photographs so that you can personalize your LO's room, even if it is for a short stay, including a calendar that shows when you will visit.
- Nurture relationships with the staff and the administration before you move your LO in.
- Prepare a copy of your most recent Family Care Plan for the facility, so that the staff can follow it as closely as possible during the transition.
- Ask for their care plan as well, so you can see how things will be different.
- Make sure everything in your LO's room works before you leave: all lights, call buzzers, television.

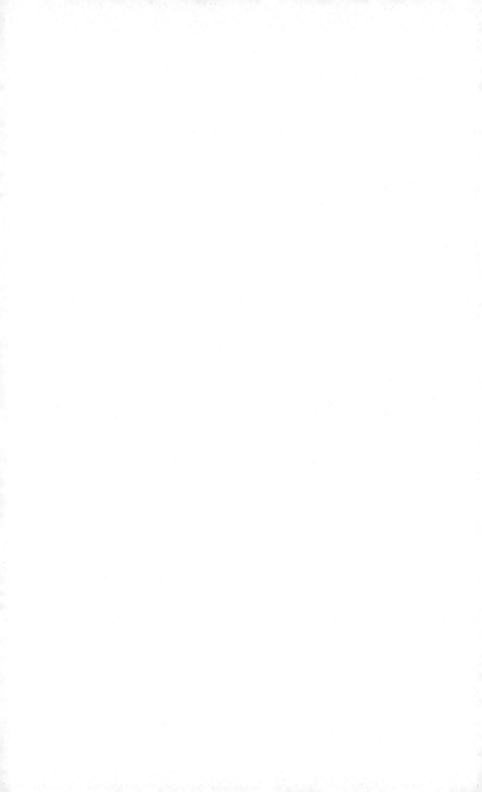

CHAPTER 11

Planning for End of Life

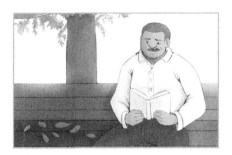

The final stages of dementia/AD can come with a mixed bag of emotions. You may feel relief that your LO will finally be in a better place or that their suffering is nearly over. You may also feel that your LO, and you for that matter, have been robbed of a contemplative passing. It's impossible to know what your LO is experiencing in the final weeks, as they will likely be nonverbal, and sleeping much of the time. Yet that doesn't mean that they aren't at peace, experiencing feelings of love of self and of others.

The hallmark of end of life for those with dementia/AD is a physical withdrawing from everyday life. This transition usually takes a few weeks and corresponds with Stage 7 of the disease. Your LO may appear to be constantly sleeping because they spend most of the day with their eyes closed. While they may not be able to speak, they can hear you and feel your loving touch.

In Stage 7, continue to provide care exactly the same way you've been doing all along even though they stay in bed all day; speak with your LO throughout the day, and identify yourself and let them know what you are going to do to help them remain comfortable before you gently do your ADL tasks. Respect their wishes when it comes to mealtime; don't force food or drink. However, keep their mouth and lips moist with disposable oral care swabs or a medicine dropper. Keep your LO clean and dry by changing their adult diapers every two hours or as needed.

You may notice that your LO's breathing has altered. It may slow down, speed up, sound shallow, or seem like there is no breathing at all for as much as a minute. You may hear a rattling sound; that occurs when they aren't swallowing the saliva building up in their throat. It sounds awful, but it doesn't mean that they are in pain. The medication atropine (1%) is an eye drop that is also often prescribed to dry secretions in the mouth to get rid of the rattling sound. Gently turning them or propping their head may help. Shifting their entire body from one side to another every 2 hours or as needed also helps prevent bedsores.

Dementia can lead to an inability to maintain a consistent body temperature, and your LO could either run a fever or feel cold/clammy. You may also notice a change in skin color. Stabilize their temperature with more blankets or fewer, and change their sleeping attire daily (this is when my T-shirt hack in Chapter 5 comes in handy), and always when they become wet. They may even appear restless, which may be a sign that they are distressed. Continue with your Daily Observation to make sure that they are not in any pain. Holding their hand may be the reassuring touch they are looking for.

At the very end, your LO may have an unexpected surge of energy. This doesn't always happen, but when it does, it is short-lived. If it does happen, take advantage of the moment, and remind your LO what you love most about them. Doing so may be healing for you, and for them.

THE STAGE 7 FAMILY CARE PLAN

When your LO is bedridden, your job is less about keeping them engaged and more about keeping them safe and comfortable. This sample schedule can be repeated every 2 hours until the end, including overnight. Throughout, you will be continuously monitoring your LO for transitioning signs, including decreasing blood pressure, breathing changes, an irregular heartbeat (which can be hard to detect), or brown, tan, or rust-colored urine. This is when your stethoscope, pulse oximeter, and blood pressure monitor will be most frequently used.

8:00 a.m.: morning ADL care: Daily Observation, bathe (sponge bath), change clothes (your LO will be wearing a limited selection of clothing at this point), provide a meal (as tolerated), resettle in bed

9:00 a.m.: read to your LO, play soft music, hold their hand, perform light massage

9:40 a.m.: check for soiled diapers, reposition your LO

10:00 a.m.: provide necessary medications for pain, agitation, and respiratory management

ARRANGE FOR HOSPICE CARE EARLY

The end-of-life transition can be difficult to attend to on your own. Fortunately, dementia/AD is one of several diagnoses that qualify for *hospice care*. This service manages the end-of-life symptoms to reduce pain and ease stress for your LO and the entire family. It is meant to improve the quality of life for your LO; many of the families that I have worked with have told me that hospice care provided them with a sense of satisfaction regarding their LO's passing. Most notably, it allows your LO to pass away with dignity outside a hospital setting.

Your LO is entitled to end-of-life hospice care as soon as their doctor believes they have a life expectancy of six months or less. The doctor orders the hospice care, which can be delivered in the home or in a skilled nursing facility. However, most families do not take full advantage of hospice care and wait until their LO is in their last week of life before asking the doctor to order it. This is a mistake, because it can provide significant support in many ways.

Your LO may also qualify for hospice, or *palliative care*, as early as Stage 5 if they are exhibiting signs of decline, particularly difficulty breathing, weight loss, or chronic pain. In this case, the same care is referred to as *palliative care* because your LO isn't on their deathbed yet. The goal of palliative care is the same as hospice: to improve your LO's overall quality of life.

Hospice/palliative care is so effective that it can actually slow the rate of decline; your LO may move in and out of hospice care several times before they pass. What's more, it is available at no cost for as long as your LO requires it; it is authorized by your LO's physician in renewable 60-day increments after an initial 90-day benefit period. Use it as a tool that provides you with hours of care that you can use as you see fit.

Hospice care is federally funded through Medicare and Medicaid, but it is managed by each state. The services can be delivered in your own home, a hospital, a nursing home, or a stand-alone hospice center. The benefits your LO will be entitled to overlap with many of the services your team is providing. However, they are filled with specialists for end-of-life care. These include the following:

- Professional medical care (doctors and nurses)
- Home health aide who specializes in hospice care
- Homemaker services (housecleaner and meal prep)
- Medical equipment (wheelchair, hospital bed)
- Medical supplies (oxygen, bandages, catheters)
- Physical, occupational, and speech/language therapists
- Dietary counseling
- Grief and counseling services
- Short-term respite care
- Prescription drugs for pain relief
- Other Medicare services related to other symptoms or conditions your LO may have

Hospice providers also have relationships with local-area clergy and will ask if you would like a pastoral visit from someone of your faith. Clergy will call and arrange for visiting times and will continue to see your LO for as long as you would like.

THE HOSPICE KIT

Whenever your LO is on hospice, they will receive a *hospice comfort kit* that is stored in the refrigerator. It contains medications for a medical crisis, which are primarily used by hospice professionals. However, these same professionals can instruct you on how to use these medications if you are alone with your LO during an emergency. Typically, the hospice intake coordinator orders the hospice kit.

A hospice kit can address:

- Anxiety
- Breathing problems

- Constipation
- Insomnia
- Nausea
- Pain

You Will Need Help at End of Life

While you may want to be the sole caregiver to your LO up through the end-of-life transition, this may not be practical or possible. As I've said, the best caregivers know when to bring in others to help them. End of life is a significant time where your LO will need extra support that you cannot provide on your own. It's a 24/7 commitment, and your LO will be better served if you can share the responsibilities.

Bringing in hospice care will allow you to have downtime, more so even than splitting the day with another family member. Familiarize yourself with exactly what your state provides so that you can make use of those benefits and create a plan that works for you.

THE POWER OF ACCEPTANCE

I once worked for a family where Benny, the patriarch, was in the last stages of dementia, and his family had been caring for him up until he was severely declining. He and his wife, Matilda, had nine kids, including a couple of nurses. Yet toward the very end of his life, they wanted me to care for their father during the night so that the family could start grieving and making funeral arrangements.

When I arrived at the house, I could tell that Benny was dying, and guessed that he would pass within the next 48 hours. However, after the second night, he was still alive. When I was getting ready to leave the next morning, I told Matilda that Benny would probably pass during the day.

By 8:00 p.m. I hadn't heard from the family, so I gave them a call. I asked how Benny was doing, and Matilda said that he was still hanging in there. I asked her if she had spent any time with him in his room that day, and she said that she had not. I suggested to her that she go in and hold his hand and talk to him.

About an hour later, I got the call: Benny was gone. Matilda had bathed him, talked to him, and 30 minutes later, he was gone. I believe that Benny wanted Matilda to be the last person he saw. He recognized his wife's touch and how she communicated with him, and realized that it was time to go.

FINAL THOUGHTS

The love and joy of caregiving are often realized at the end of a good day. In that quiet space, you realize that you have given your best. You have done all the right things for your LO to have a successful day. That feeling of accomplishment can be felt right to the very end, even when your LO can no longer share how they feel. Somehow, you will know.

My hope for you is that you can approach your LO each morning calmly, and by the end of the day have had a positive moment worth recording in your binder. It could be that your LO had a good laugh, or that they finished every meal, or that they were able to complete the exercise routine. As you tally your wins, you'll quickly see that you are an excellent caregiver.

Every day there will be challenges, and you are now ready to face them. You have done the hard work of preparing for all scenarios and have proactively looked at what is happening now, and what is coming for the future. And with a clear mind, you have fully transitioned from denial to acceptance.

ACKNOWLEDGMENTS

This book has been a long time coming, and I'm so very grateful to so many people for helping me on this journey.

I want to thank my family. My husband, Ronald, has been my rock ever since we were teenagers. He has always supported whatever I've wanted to do. My children, Ronald Christopher and Regann Marie, along with my grandson, Royce, my brothers, and my nieces and nephews have watched me evolve. I love you all!

Beyond my immediate family, my aunts, uncles, cousins, and in-laws are like a second family. Dorothy Nicholas was the first nurse I met when I was four years old. She helped raise me and is like a second mom. My great-aunt Gladys was the first nurse in our family and inspired me to become one. My cousin Donna Knapper and I are the third generation of nurses. Takeisha Davis, MD, MPH, my cousin's daughter, has upped our family game and is the CEO for New Orleans East Hospital.

Then there is Pamela Liflander. I believe that there are no such things as coincidences, and meeting Pam proves my point. We were two strangers sitting next to each other at a Columbia Business School Alumni event, attending for very different reasons. Yet we had in common a fondness for interviewing new people. Within 5 minutes I learned that she was a former book editor with a book idea, looking for a subject expert. I turned out to be exactly the woman she was looking for: a home-care expert who was also thinking about writing a book. Our relationship over the four years it has taken to write this book has been like no other friendship I've had. And in the end, she helped me find my voice and put my words on the page.

My agent, Carol Mann, has believed in this project from the start, and found us a dream team at Avery. My editor, Nina Shield, and her group, including Hannah Steigmeyer, Marlena Brown, and Victoria Adamo, along with my copyeditor, Amy Schneider, and proofreaders, Patricia Callahan and Erica Rose, have helped us create a book that in every way lives up to its potential. I was so fortunate to meet and have the expert read of Adrienne Ingrum, who reviewed the proposal to make sure that I was true to my experience and my community. Illustrator Gregory Jones Jr. infused our artwork with his own experiences with caring for a loved one with dementia. And thank you, thank you to Nikki Kimbrough, fitness expert and personal trainer to the stars, for creating two awesome workouts just for this book.

I have also had enormous support and help from my colleagues who reviewed the manuscript, shared their own experiences, and helped me better understand and express my own. These include David Stevens, MD, MPH, Mark Borg Jr., PhD, and Sarah Jean-Baptiste, LPN. Pamela Macon and my cousin Deshonda Charles Smith, Esq., shared their knowledge about estate and end-of-life planning. Jacqueline Wallace, a retired Social Security representative, explained how government benefits work. Zina Lee and Melanie Felton shared their knowledge of "board and care" homes; Lisa Smith, PhD, helped me understand how integral physical therapy is for at-home care. Sheila Franklin shared her knowledge regarding health insurance companies and benefits. Carolyn McLauren is a speech-language pathologist who helped me with the instructions for swallowing. And thanks to my home-care nursing friends: Karen Ford, Geraldine Sinceno, Bonnette Bryant, Lydia Wicks, Lisa Nelson, Laura Alvarez, Jason Bauer, Barbara Kirksey, and Laquisha Jones, my grandson's mother. My social workers Martha Sanchez and Lillian Serrano were very helpful. Olivia Francis Webber, a former elementary school principal, invited me to education conferences, and teachers Sonia Farr and Paige Cragg were great sounding boards for the activities section.

I want to mention all my friends who have supported me over the years and shared their dementia/AD experiences with me: Donna Anderson Tookes, Agneta Brewster Ballestros, Yvette Cochrane, Nicole Kearney, Candice Sanchez McFarlane, Sharon Taylor Simmons Brown, Olive Cooper, Shelley Jallow, PhD, Terri Smith, Denise Galiber, Diana Quarles, and Peter Obermeyer.

I have to thank the people who make me look good. Makeup artists Torya Strother and Angela Middleton set me up for success with photographer Earl Anderson. And my social media consultant, Jonathan Logan, and my public speaking coach, DeLores Pressley, are preparing me for promoting my work.

Lastly, I want to thank the Alzheimer's Association, which has embraced my home care work and my advocacy. I'm particularly indebted to Debbie Warburton of the New York State Coalition, who invited me to join their state and federal delegations. They do important work for all of our futures, and I'm thrilled to be part of it.

AARP: www.aarp.org

Alzheimer's Association: www.alz.org

Nikki Kimbrough videos: www.getfitwithnik.com/caregiving
-with-love-joy

Cannabis resources: www.justanswer.com, www.ezdoctor.com,
and www.amwell.com

Medicare: www.medicare.gov

Meals on Wheels: www.mealsonwheelsamerica.org

NOTES

Chapter 1: Is This Behavior Normal? Accepting the New Reality

1. Alzheimer's Association, "2019 Alzheimer's Disease Facts and Figures," *Alzheimer's & Dementia* 15 (2019): 321–387. https://doi.org/10.1016/j.jalz.2019.01.010.

2. AARP and National Alliance for Caregiving, *Caregiving in the U.S. 2020* (Washington, DC: AARP, May 2020). https://doi.org/10.26419-2Fppi.00103.001.

Chapter 2: Becoming the Best Caregiver

1. Jon LaPook, "Following a Couple from Diagnosis to the Final Stages of Alzheimer's," *60 Minutes*, August 12, 2018. https://www.cbsnews.com/news/60-minutes-alzheimers-disease-following-a-couple-from-diagnosis-to-the-final-stages/.

2. Jane E. Brody, "Alzheimer's? Your Paperwork May Not Be in Order," *New York Times*, April 30, 2018. https://www.nytimes.com/2018/04/30/well/live/an-advance-directive-for-patients-with-dementia.html.

3. J. K. Rao et al., "Completion of Advance Directives among U.S. Consumers," *American Journal of Preventive Medicine* 46, 1 (2014): 65–70.

Chapter 3: Self-Care Strategies: Taking Care of the Caregiver

1. R. Plutchik, "A General Psychoevolutionary Theory of Emotion," in R. Plutchik and H. Kellerman (eds.), *Emotion: Theory, Research and Experience, Theories of Emotion*, vol. 1 (New York: Academic Press, 1980), pp. 3–33.

Chapter 4: Organizing the Home

1. Christopher F. Schuetze, "Take a Look at These Unusual Strategies for Fighting Dementia," *New York Times*, August 22, 2018. https://www.nytimes.com/2018/08/22/world/europe/dementia-care-treatment-symptoms-signs.html.

Chapter 6: Filling the Family Care Plan with Appropriate Activities

1. C. L. Williams and R. M. Tappen, "Exercise Training for Depressed Older Adults with Alzheimer's Disease," *Aging and Mental Health* 12, 1 (2008): 72–80. https://doi.org/10.1080/13607860701529932.

2. V. E. Sturm et al., "Big Smile, Small Self: Awe Walks Promote Prosocial Positive Emotions in Older Adults," *Emotion* (2009), advance online publication. https://doi.org/10.1037/emo0000876.

Chapter 7: Dealing with Difficult Behaviors

1. Debra Fulghum Bruce, "Drugs That Cause Depression," WebMD, March 8, 2021. https://www.webmd.com/depression/guide/medicines-cause-depression.

2. S. Petersen et al., "The Utilization of Robotic Pets in Dementia Care," *Journal of Alzheimer's Disease* 55, 2 (2017): 569–574. https://doi.org/10.3233/JAD-160703.

3. Amy Clare et al., "Using Music to Develop a Multisensory Communicative Environment for People with Late-Stage Dementia." *Gerontologist* 60, 6 (2020): 1115–1125. https://doi.org/10.1093/geront/gnz169.

Chapter 8: Identifying and Treating Common Medical Problems

1. "Alzheimer's: Managing Sleep Problems," Mayo Clinic, December 21, 2019. https://www.mayoclinic.org/healthy-lifestyle/caregivers/in-depth/alzheimers/art-20047832.

Chapter 10: Coordinating Respite Care

1. Alzheimer's Association, "2021 Alzheimer's Disease Facts and Figures, Special Report: Race, Ethnicity and Alzheimer's in America," *Alzheimer's & Dementia* 17, 3 (2021). https://www.alz.org/media/Documents/alzheimers-facts-and-figures.pdf.

INDEX

scheduling appropriate activities,
151–93. *See also* activity scheduling
stress and, 32–33. *See also* self-care
strategies
team approach to, 33–55, 136. *See also*
Family Care Plan
retrogenesis (return to childhood), 13
reversible memory loss, 15–17
risk awareness, 8
risperidone (Risperdal), 205, 236
Ritalin (methylphenidate), 236
rivastigmine (Exelon), 236
robotic therapy pets and dolls, 207, 208
rooms. *See also specific rooms*
color choices for, 98–99, 109
organization, 100–110
rugs, 96
rummage boxes, 168

scheduling appropriate activities. *See*
activity scheduling
seasonal allergies, 221
self-care strategies, 57–90
about, 57
burnout prevention, 117, 151, 226
community connections, 88–89
eating healthfully, 59–61
emotion management, 86–88
exercise routine, 61–78, 273
hobbies, 83–84
meditation, 78–80
relationship with Loved One,
84–85
scheduling using the Family Care Plan,
58–59
sleep hygiene, 80–83
spa day, 59
stigmatization issues, 88–89, 90
support groups, 89, 90
self-soothing, 200
senior grants, 96
sensory boxes, 168
Seroquel (quetiapine), 236

sertraline (Zoloft), 236
shades, for windows, 99–100
short-term residential program, 252,
253–54
shower equipment and setup,
109–10, 114
showering, 138–40
Sinequan, 230–31
60 Minutes, 33
skilled nursing inpatient facility (nursing
home), xiii, 252–59
skills for caregiving
for ADLs, 117–50. *See also* activities of
daily living
dealing with difficult behaviors,
195–212. *See also specific behaviors*
dealing with medical problems, 213–37.
See also specific medical problems
for eating and mealtimes, 239–50. *See
also* mealtimes
skin issues and care, 122–23, 138–40, 141,
216, 219–20, 222–25
sleep hygiene, 13, 80–83, 203, 210,
225–31, 236
socialization opportunities, 41, 153, 158
Social Security, 47
social worker, 39
sodium valproate (Depakote), 236
soothing behaviors, 200
sorority chapter resources, 89
spatial and visual awareness, 8
specialist providers, 37–38
speech and communication difficulties,
209–10
statins, 204
stigma of dementia, 88–89, 90
stimulants, 236
stress, 32–33. *See also* self-care strategies
sundowning, 20, 210–11
supplemental care provider, 40
Supplemental Security Income, 47
supplements, 230, 247, 250
support groups, 89, 90

Printed in Great Britain
by Amazon

33133900R00172